# The Ultimate TMJ Guide

**Published by Cleal Publishing**

**Copyright © 2017 Cleal Publishing**

**Legal & Disclaimer**

The information contained in this book is not designed to replace or take the place of any form of medicine or professional medical advice. The information in this book has been provided for educational and entertainment purposes only.

The information contained in this book has been compiled from sources deemed reliable, and it is accurate to the best of the Author's knowledge; however, the Author or Publisher cannot guarantee its accuracy and validity and cannot be held liable for any errors or omissions. Changes are periodically made to this book. You must consult your doctor or get professional medical advice before using any of the suggested remedies, techniques, or information in this book.

Upon using the information contained in this book, you agree to hold harmless the Author from and against any damages, costs, and expenses, including any legal fees potentially resulting from the application of any of the information provided by this guide. This disclaimer applies to any damages or injury caused by the use and application, whether directly or indirectly, of any advice or information presented, whether for breach of contract, tort, negligence, personal injury, criminal intent, or under any other cause of action.

You agree to accept all risks of using the information presented inside this book. You need to consult a professional medical practitioner in order to ensure you are both able and healthy enough to participate in this program.

# Table of Contents

# Introduction

The TMJ disorder, also known as temporomandibular joint disorder is seen very often in dentist checkups. They call it "having TMJ," which means a painful TM joint. When this joint is not functioning normally and gives pain with movement, it is called temporomandibular disorder or TM dysfunction. It is sometimes also referred to as "myofascial pain disorder."

The main causes include anything related to the jaw, such as injury to the teeth or the misalignment of teeth during the developmental phase or growth. It can also be caused by habitual grinding of teeth without having anything in the mouth, poor posture, anxiety, arthritis of the joint, or excessive chewing of the gum.

TMD is a mixture of different conditions as a complex rather than a single condition. About one-fifth of the general population is affected by TMD. Most of these are people aged between 25 and 50. *It is the most common cause of painful facial region pain due to dental causes.*

The condition itself may not be serious at all but the symptoms it can cause (such as pain in the jaws, clicking of the jaw joint, or popping) can be extremely troublesome. It is, therefore, necessary to address this issue seriously to avoid the symptoms and possible complications in future.

This is eBook will be your friend. We will walk you through the TMJ basics all the way to curative techniques and self-management options.

Keep reading to learn more.

# Section A: The basics

# Chapter 1: Understanding TMJ

## What is TMJ?

TMJ, also known as the temporomandibular joint, is one of the most important joints in the body. It is located in the facial region on both the right and left sides. This joint is responsible for jaw movement and for attachment of the lower part of the face to the skull.

The TMJs are simply the jaw joints on either side of the head, in front of the ears. These joints provide motion, allowing you to open or close your mouth when you eat or speak. The joint is created between mandible bone and temporal bone.

If you want to feel the joint movements, you can do it by placing your fingers on the ear and opening your mouth. Both of these TMJs are flexible, so they can move in the up, down, forward, and backward directions, enabling us to talk and chew without any difficulty.

The TMJ is prone to certain injuries and traumas as a result of blows from the sides. Moreover, they can also be strained by muscular injuries or dental injuries, thus causing painful TMJ.

## Anatomical background of normal jaw and TMJ

The TMJs are located right in front of the ears and they can be found by placing your fingers in front of the ears. You can feel the upper part of the lower jaw by opening it while your fingers are placed over it. The upper bone of the TMJ is a part of the temporal bone and the lower portion is part of the lower jaw, or mandible.

Between these two bones in the TMJ is a cushion that slides between the bones as you move your jaw up or down. There are a lot of muscles in the joint that control its movements in all directions, providing a vast diversion of mobility. The disc of the joint is also controlled by a ligament that is located in the back of joint. Surrounding the whole joint is a capsule containing a fluid that lubricates the joint to help prevent injuries due to movement of the joint. In addition to this, blood supply and nerves that supply the joint with nourishment and sensation.

## Why is TMJ important?

Both of these joints (i.e., the left and right TMJs) are complexes of dual functional joints, as they serve both as hinges and as sliding joints. This movement of the jaw helps in a wide variety of functions.

Fully opened, the jaw is about 40 to 50 millimeters for adults, as measured from the lower front teeth to the edge of upper front teeth. During jaw movements, only the mandible, the lower part of the jaw, moves.

When the mouth is open, the rounded end of the lower jaw (the condyle) slides along the temporal part of the joint and these joints move back to their normal positions when the mouth is closed. The disc in the joint absorbs shocks imparted to the jaw during its function.

These functions altogether make this a very important joint in eating, talking, and yawning.

# Different types of TMJ disorders

There are wide varieties of TMJ disorders that can affect the jaw joint and the muscles associated with the joint, called the chewing muscles or muscles of mastication. All of these disorders fall into three main categories:

☐ Pain in the muscles that control jaw movements; this is called myofascial pain.

☐ Internal derangement of the joint that includes a displaced disk or a jaw dislocated or condylar injury.

☐ Lastly, there are conditions that can cause inflammatory and degenerative processes affecting the temporomandibular joint, referred to as arthritis.

A person may sometimes have more than one of these conditions or complications at the same time as an overlapping presentation. There can also be some other health problems associated with the TMJ disorders; for example, chronic fatigue disorder or sleep problems, even fibromyalgia, which is a very painful condition affecting the muscles and the soft tissues all over the body. All of these disorders may share some common symptoms that suggest having a similar underlying mechanism. However, it might not be true that they all have a common cause.

Problems such as a rheumatic disease, especially arthritis, may also cause pain in the TMJ as a secondary condition. Rheumatic diseases include a larger group of disorders that cause inflammation, pain, and stiffness in the joints, the bones, and muscles all over the body. Arthritis and TMJ disorders may involve inflammation of the tissues that line the joints. The exact mechanism and relation between these conditions are not very well known.

Jaw joint and muscle disorders cause temporomandibular syndrome, but the mechanism behind it is still unknown. What is truly known is that these symptoms worsen over time. Most of the population is affected by a mild form of this disorder. Their symptoms and conditions may improve significantly or may even disappear spontaneously due to other underlying causes, such as those associated with dental issues or problems associated with the ear. For others, the condition may be chronic and long-term with persistent and constant excruciating pain.

## Causes of TMJ disorder

There can be many causes of a TMJ disorder but some of the main ones should be noticed and evaluated for timely management. Trauma or blows to the joint play a huge role in some of the disorders of TMJ, but for most joint and muscles problem (such as myopathy), clinicians don't know the actual cause. This condition is more common in women than in men, so efforts are being made to link the conditions somehow to the female hormones affecting the TMJ.

For most people, the symptoms might resolve spontaneously without any reason, in which instance, it can be safely said that the cause may have been a bad bite or orthodontic braces, which can trigger a TMJ disorder. Moreover, there are some scientific studies claiming that habits like teeth-grinding or clicking of the jaw joint lead to serious problems. On the contrary, jaw sounds are common in the general population. Jaw noises alone, without pain or limited jaw movement, do not indicate a TMJ disorder and do not warrant treatment.

## Signs and symptoms

A variety of signs and symptoms can be linked to TMJ disorder, with the help of which one can diagnose him/her self with this disorder. Any kind of pain, most particularly in the upper chewing muscles or the jaw joint, is one of the most common symptoms of TMJ disorder. Other symptoms linked to TMJ disorder are:

- ☐ Pain radiating to the face or the neck including the jaw

- ☐ Stiffness of jaw muscles

- ☐ Pain with movements of the jaw and/or limited movement of jaw that can cause 'locking of jaw'

- ☐ Clicking becomes painful, along with popping or grating in the jaw joint when the mouth is opened or closed

- ☐ A change in the way upper and lower teeth were fitting together

## Possible complications of TMJ

For most people with a TMJ disorder, the condition can be managed without any effects or impact on life. When left untreated, however, the TMJ can lead to chronic conditions of everlasting pain and recurrent headache episodes, along with other adverse effects.

The complications of TMJ disorder and how they act depend largely on the cause of the condition. Simply put, most symptoms of TMJ can cause stress on mental health, along with the health of the joint. These can cause denervation of the joint and may also affect nerves and vessels in the path of the joint or those directly supplying the joint.

11

Although TMJ is not a life-threatening condition, if it is left untreated, the negative effects of TMJ disorder can affect your quality of life over time and pain becomes more miserable as the condition gradually worsens.

One of the most widely reported and seen complications of TMJ is clicking of the jaw. Research has discovered that about two-thirds of patients who developed painless clicking of the jaw at the start later developed painful clicking of the jaw joint. Other conditions that can become a complication of TMJ later in life include intense headaches, pain in the neck, back or shoulder region, and ringing in the ears (also known as tinnitus). This can also be accompanied by pain in the ear.

# Chapter 2: Diagnosing the issue

## Diagnosis of TMJ

The patient's history, such as pain location, duration, onset, and aggravating factors of the problem will help you diagnose a TMJ disorder. A physical exam in which you can elicit joint noises, masticatory muscle softness, and limited mandible functions will help narrow down the list of possible diseases, and further investigations will confirm the diagnosis.

It must be noted that patients may present one symptom or a combination of symptoms. It is, therefore, necessary to develop a solid approach toward the correct diagnosis.

## Risk factors

A risk factor increases the likelihood of getting a disease or condition. It is possible to develop TMJ syndrome with or without the risk factors listed below. However, the more risk factors there are, the greater the likelihood of developing TMJ syndrome. If you have a number of risk factors, ask y healthcare provider what you can do to reduce your risk.

Risk factors for TMJ syndrome include, but are not limited to, the following:

### Stress

Individuals experiencing a lot of stress in their lives may have an increased risk of TMJ syndrome. Some of the stress-related habits that may increase your risk of TMJ syndrome include:

- ☐ Habitually clenching and unclenching your jaw
- ☐ Grinding your teeth during the day and/or at night in your sleep

☐ Constantly or very regularly chewing things, such as gum or ice, for long periods of time

## Medical conditions

The following medical conditions may increase your risk of TMJ syndrome:

☐ Misaligned teeth or misaligned bite

☐ Jaw or facial deformities

☐ Arthritic conditions, such as:

    o Osteoarthritis

    o Rheumatoid arthritis

☐ Synovitis (inflammation of the membrane that lines the TMJ)

☐ History of jaw or facial injuries (such as fractures or dislocations of the jaw or mandible)

## Age

Most people report TMJ syndrome symptoms between the ages of 30 and 50.

Ill-fitting dentures or poorly fitted dentures are thought to be a risk factor for TMJ syndrome, particularly in this age.

## Female gender

TMJ affects twice as many women as men, and female hormones may be the possible cause. Many studies show that estrogen receptors in the knee joint and estradiol levels in synovial fluid correlate with the severity of osteoarthritis. Once full-flown osteoarthritis has developed, it soon affects the TMJ, too. Other studies link an increase in estradiol level in both women and men with TMJ syndrome, while another study found an inverse correlation between circulating estrogen and joint pain. Overall, there is inadequate evidence supporting the correlation between TMJ syndrome and the level of female hormones.

## Depression and anxiety

Depression is a risk factor to TMJ since it correlates with chronic pain syndromes. A study indicated that severely depressed individuals are at higher risk for an onset of TMJ syndrome than non-depressed persons.

# Key factors

## Cyclic pain

Patients experiencing myofascial pain and dysfunctional cyclic pain in the tooth from brushing at nighttime generally develop TMJ syndrome in the long run. Furthermore, pain is highly common with osteoarthritis patients and, if it is associated with using the jaw, then is most likely due to TMJ syndrome.

## Prolonged pain

Internal anatomical derangement of the joint causes an unremitting pain that causes and worsens with TMJ syndrome.

## Joint noise

Myofascial pain and dysfunction symptoms include palpable or audible joint click in the jaw area as it opens and closes. Patients with internal derangement have a clicking and possible locking of the jaw. Osteoarthritis is often accompanied by joint crepitus. All these different kinds of noises indicate possible joint disorder, which is most likely diagnosed as TMJ disorder.

### Abnormal mandibular movement

The maximum mandibular opening is 42 to 55 mm in a normal individual. With an incurring problem, the movement may be reduced to <35mm. Such patients usually complain that their teeth lock or they have a bad feeling while biting due to an uncorrected deviation from the maximal mouth opening.

### Masticatory muscle tenderness

Upon maximal mouth opening, the muscles of mastication are tender to palpation with pain and soreness.

### Other risk factors

There is some evidence that women taking hormone replacement therapy are more likely to develop symptoms of TMJ, as several studies have shown a link between TMJ syndrome and female hormonal imbalance. Hormone replacement therapy results in estrogen changes that modulate the functions of the nervous, skeletal, and immune system in ways that are likely to cause TMJ disorders.

## Psychological factors

Emotional, behavioral, and interpersonal relationships play an etiological role in TMJ disorders by eliciting muscle tensions and different oral habits. Some studies indicate that psychological factors such as stress and anxiety induce muscular hyperactivity and fatigue. Furthermore, these factors cause muscle spasms, which lead to contracture and degenerative arthritis. Therefore, physiological factors are quite related to TMJ cases.

## Malocclusion

In the past, adjustment of occlusion was a form of treatment for TMJ syndrome. The National Institutes of Health does not support this method since no study has ever established a link between malocclusion and TMJ syndrome.

## Headache, backache, earache, or neck pain

A history of headaches, backache, earache, or neck pain is also a likely cause of TMJ disorder, especially if the pain is chronic and is not properly managed over time.

# Diagnosis of TMJ

There is no extensively approved standard test currently available for diagnosing TMJ disorders. The diagnosis of TMJ osteoarthritis is also difficult due to other TMJ pathologies that present analogous aspects to clinical and radiographic techniques. The diagnostic process involves a description of the patient's symptoms, details of past medical and dental history, and examination of the problem areas, including the head, neck, face, and jaw. Another appropriate decisive factor useful in ruling out TMJ identification disorders is facial pain, which indicates divergent conditions such as ear infections, sinusitis, headaches, and facial nerve pains.

A TMJ clinical examination is the tool commonly used to identify symptoms. However, imaging TMJs is applicable for more detailed information. The diagnostic procedure involves assessing the temperature of the skin, muscle rupture, swelling, reference points, and trigger locations. Temporomandibular joint dysfunction affects a majority of the population unknowingly, and some of the notable clinical symptoms include: pain around the region of TMJ, prolonged headaches, muscle tenderness, earaches, noises around the joint, such as clicking, popping, or grating, incomplete opening or mandible deviation in opening/closing, locking, and changes in occlusion due to altered mandible positioning.

## Imaging

The TMJ assessment approach entails evaluating patient history as well as clinical examination. Normally, the clinical examination results are sufficient for medical practitioners to determine preliminary diagnosis and treatment. However, for advanced diagnosis, imaging of TMJ is paramount for detailed information that is not available from the clinical examination.

Imaging assists in the diagnosis of TMJ when history and physical examination results are equivocal. Even though uncommonly used, multiple imaging modalities are available to obtain extra information about the suspected TMD etiologies.

Furthermore, TMJ imaging is employed when the following indications are noted: Normal treatment is ineffective or deterioration of symptoms, patients with a history of trauma, significant dysfunction, patients with abnormalities of the sensory and motor system, unusual occlusion changes such as osseous abnormality, or suspicion of infection. Moreover, TMJ imaging is applicable if a patient has a history of TMJ and has never enrolled in a treatment plan that involves extensive reconstructive work or orthodontia. Such a treatment plan usually alters the occlusion, thus predisposing patients to recurrences of TMD symptoms. Nevertheless, the imaging process enables dentists to assess the integrity and establish associations of TMJ osseous components, ascertain the degree of progress of the disease, and appraise the impacts of treatment. For proper diagnosis, the patient's history and clinical findings should be linked with imaging results to enhance effective plan of treatment.

## Choice of imaging technique

The choice of imaging technique for TMJ depends on the explicit clinical problems, such as soft and hard tissues to be imaged, the dose of radiation, the cost, and available diagnosis information. Furthermore, advancements in technology, i.e., the reduction in radiation doses and improvement in imaging, the enabling of hard tissues and evaluation of osseous contours, establishing a positional correlation between the glenoid fossa and the condyle, and determining the range of motion. On the other hand, images of the soft tissues are determined if more information regarding the disk position and structure or abnormalities around the soft tissues are required. Ideally, such images should capture the whole joint and surrounding structures in a minimum of two planes perpendicular to each other, i.e., lateral and frontal planes. An additional orientation is also significant since it enables three-dimension evaluation of the joint.

## Panoramic radiography

Panoramic radiography is also called a "screening" projection. This type of radiography is used to project pictures of the TMJ; however, it must be combined with other hard tissue imaging techniques. Furthermore, panoramic radiography provides a general image of the jaws and teeth, thus allowing assessment of mandible symmetry, the dentition, and the maxillary sinuses. Clinically, mandible asymmetry might not produce a clear view; however, divergence in the size of one condyle or one side of the mandible is a causative factor in the development of TMD.

19

Odontogenic inflammatory disease, especially in the posterior end of the maxillary teeth, creates pain in the TMJ, hence reproducing TMD. Panoramic views of abnormality in the teeth should be imaged in one or more intra-oral views to enhance maximum bony details and arrive at a precise diagnosis. However, caution should be taken while interpreting the radiographic appearances of the TMJs in a panoramic view; for example, positions of the condylar ends cannot be assessed, since the patient is usually placed in a protrusive and slightly open position. Nevertheless, images of glenoid fossa are not clear and condyle articulating surfaces are distorted due to the projection angle. Therefore, osseous components of the joints cannot be precisely evaluated using this imaging technique.

## Cephalometric radiography

Cephalometric radiographs are significant accessories in the TMJ imaging study. This film radiograph is more useful in patients with neoplasm/cancer of the jaw area, fractures of the condylar necks, or developmental abnormalities.

## Tomography

Tomography is quite instrumental in imaging TMJ since it can be done using conventional or computed tomography. Furthermore, it has replaced traditional plain film techniques, i.e., trans-cranial and trans-pharyngeal views, since it has the advantage of illustrating the TMJs in thin layers or slice augmentation. Since the source of x-rays and the film are in motion, they are capable of blurring structures that are not predetermined to be on the plane of focus. Moreover, imaging the joints at diverse orientations helps to produce views that are perpendicular to each other.

# Conventional tomography

Using conventional tomography, the area of interest moves through the plane of focus, thus making several exposures. Angulations of the condylar head are viewed using the submentovertex axis in order to rectify the angulation of tomographic images. This method creates an undistorted view of joint morphology, which enables correct evaluation of the condylar position.

Occasionally, several image slices in the lateral and frontal plane are made, so the sagittal images contain information on the condylar position with respect to the glenoid fossa, which can be taken to various positions in the mandibles. The more common view is the sagittal, which exposes the teeth in the maximum length with the utmost open position. However, an additional view with a splint in place may also be taken. A frontal image enables evaluation of the condylar and glenoid fossa morphology in the mediolateral orientation and this view is quite significant in identifying erosive changes of the articular surfaces. The technique is time-consuming and images are inherently blurred due to superimposition of various neighboring structures on the image at the plane of the interest.

# Diagnostic injections

Injections of local anesthetic at the trigger point involving the muscles of mastication can be a diagnostic adjunct to distinguish the source of the jaw pain. The procedure should be performed only by a physician or dentist with much experience in anesthetizing the auriculotemporal nerve region. If well performed, the complication rate is very low. Moreover, persistent pain after appropriate nerve blockage should alert the clinician to re-evaluate TMD symptoms and consider an alternative diagnosis.

## Ultrasound

Ultrasound is a useful diagnostic tool, especially for preliminary assessment of the disc displacement. High-resolution ultrasonography provides a sensitivity of 69% in the detection of internal derangements of TMJ. Furthermore, high-resolution ultrasound provides a greater advantage during investigation since it allows viewing of the articular disk during the mouth opening movement. The principle behind ultrasonography relies on ultrasonic sound waves produced by the transducer, which travel through the TMJ and are reflected on transiting through disparate anatomical structures. The reflected sound is then read by the same emitting device and is later translated into images.

## MRI

Positive ultrasound findings of the disc's displacement should be confirmed with MRI.

# Differential diagnosis

The differential diagnosis for TMJ is listed below.TMJ disorders cause displaced pain and headaches. Some studies project that 55 percent of the patients referred to neurologists have significant symptoms of TMJ disorders.

| Disease/ Condition | Differentiating Signs/Symptoms | Differentiating Tests |
|---|---|---|
| Sinusitis | Sinusitis pain is localized to the paranasal and frontal sinuses. Pain from sinusitis is usually worse when bending forward.<br><br>TMJ syndrome usually involves the TMJ region and possibly the temporal regions. | Otoscopic examination may reveal an abnormality, such as an effusion or obstruction in the ear cavity.<br><br>Evaluation is best performed by a dentist when dental pathology is suspected. |
| Pericoronitis | Joint clicking is absent; breath may be malodorous; pericoronal tissues may be inflamed and erythematous. | Examination reveals mandibular posterior teeth (especially third molars) are erupting. |
| Chronic headache | Joint clicking is absent; pain is not cyclic. | There are no differentiating tests |
| Dental pain | Hot/cold testing of teeth indicates extreme sensitivity.<br><br>Tapping the tooth elicits pain.<br><br>Joint clicking is absent | Dental x-rays may reveal periapical pathology.<br><br>Evaluation is best performed by a dentist when dental pathology is suspected. |

| SLE | Clinical manifestations of SLE may be present, including malar rash or discoid lupus (thick, red, scaly patches on the skin).<br><br>Small joints of the hand and wrist are usually affected, although any joint is at risk.<br><br>Other presenting features include pericarditis, myocarditis, and endocarditis; pulmonary manifestations; autoimmune hepatitis; and glomerulonephritis. | Markers of systemic disease: anemia, thrombocytopenia, neutropenia, deranged liver function tests.<br><br>Positive antinuclear antibody and anti-extractable nuclear antigen on serological testing. |
|---|---|---|
| Rheumatoid arthritis | Patients with rheumatoid arthritis may have other joint involvement, particularly symmetrical small joint polyarthritis in | In rheumatoid arthritis, ESR and C-reactive protein (CRP) are abnormal and rheumatoid factor and anti-cyclic |

| | | |
|---|---|---|
| | the hands, chiefly affecting the metatarsophalangeal joints and sparing the distal interphalangeal joints.<br><br>Patients with acute rheumatoid arthritis may also feel generally ill with fatigue and low mood. | citrullinated (anti-CCP) antibodies are positive.<br><br>Typical rheumatoid arthritis erosive changes are seen on x-ray, MRI, or ultrasound. |
| Giant cell arteritis | Patients typically have pain and tenderness over the temporal artery, which may occur with amaurosis fugax and loss of vision.<br><br>Pain resolves within three days of high-dose corticosteroid treatment. | Duplex scanning of temporal arteries may reveal thickening of the arterial wall.<br><br>Sedimentation rate >100 mm/hour.<br><br>CRP is usually elevated.<br><br>Biopsy shows giant cell arteritis. |
| Neuralgias | Joint clicking is usually absent.<br><br>Facial pain is elicited by touching a trigger point. | Clinical diagnosis. |

# When to see a doctor?

A physician or dentist should be contacted in case of injury to the jaw or the face, and:

- ☐ When the jaw is painful,

- ☐ If the jaw is locked open or shut, or you are unable to move your jaw easily or smoothly; this may be a sign of disc displacement, dislocation, or fracture.

- ☐ When the jaw appears to be deformed or swollen.

- ☐ When there is a swelling in the sides of the face.

- ☐ When the teeth no longer fit together as usual when biting down (malocclusion).

- ☐ In case of severe headache or when neck ache strikes suddenly, without apparent cause, or is different from previous headaches.

- ☐ Pain when moving your jaw, i.e., biting, chewing, swallowing, talking, yawning, etc., that does not get better after two weeks of home treatment.

- ☐ Anxiety, stress, or work-related problems causing jaw discomfort and pain.

- ☐ Continued symptoms, such as a clicking or cracking sound or jaw locks after two weeks of home treatments.

# Section B: Management and treatment
# Chapter 3: Management Options
## Finding the right healthcare provider

TMD symptoms require a medical doctor to rule out some of the conditions that may mimic TMJ. For example, facial pain can be a symptom of many conditions, such as sinus or ear infections, decayed or abscessed teeth, various types of headache, facial neuralgia (nerve-related facial pain), and even tumors. Other diseases, such as Ehlers-Danlos syndrome, dystonia, Lyme disease, and scleroderma may also affect the function of the TMJ, hence warranting a suitable healthcare provider. Symptoms such as infrequent pain in the jaw joint or tenderness of the chewing muscles in the jaw are ordinary and may not be of much concern. However, if the pain is severe or persistent, it is recommended that you see a doctor. One should also see a healthcare professional if it hurts to open and close the jaw or if one has difficulty in swallowing food. TMJ treatment at an early stage is recommended if the condition is identified as soon as possible. Early identification enables the doctor to explain the functioning of the joints and offer self-care tips, such as breaking poor habits that may aggravate the joint or facial pain.

Identification of qualified TMJ healthcare providers in the past has proven to be a tedious process. However, there is no medical or dental specialty of qualified experts trained in the care and treatment of TMD. As a result, there are no established standards of care in clinical practice. Although a variety of healthcare providers advertise themselves as "TMJ specialists," more than

50 different treatments available today are not based on scientific evidence. These doctors practice according to one of many different schools of thought on how to best treat TMD. This means that you, the patient, may have difficulty finding the right care.

However, the first step is education about TMJ. Informed patients are better able to communicate with healthcare providers, ask questions, and make knowledgeable decisions.

Second, the National Institute of Health (NIH) advises patients to look for a healthcare provider who understands musculoskeletal disorders (affecting muscles, bones, and joints) and who is trained in treating pain conditions. Moreover, pain clinics, hospitals, and universities are often a good source of advice, particularly when pain becomes chronic and interferes with daily life. Patients might first be diagnosed with TMJ by a primary-care provider (PCP), such as a family practitioner, internist, or a child's pediatrician. A doctor may refer you to an oral and maxillofacial expert, an otolaryngologist (also called a nose, ear, and throat doctor or an ENT specialist), or a dentist who specializes in jaw disorders (prosthodontist, also called a prosthetic dentist) for further treatment. Patients might also see a pain-management specialist if TMJ pain is severe.

Complex cases, often marked by chronic and severe pain, jaw dysfunction, comorbid conditions, and diminished quality of life, will likely require a team of doctors from fields such as neurology, rheumatology, pain management, and other specialties for diagnosis and treatment.

# Self-care tips

- Rest the muscles and joints. This enhances healing, and it includes:

    o A soft food diet — refrain from consuming crunchy and chewy foods, such as nuts, chips, carrots, and hard bread.

    o Avoid chewing gum.

    o Avoid clenching, i.e., learn to keep teeth apart, face and jaw relaxed. This simple step relaxes the tense and taut muscles and promotes healing of damage to temporomandibular joints. "Lips together and teeth apart" is important advice to break the daytime habit of clenching and/or grinding teeth. This process enhances separation of the teeth and simultaneously relaxing the jaw and facial muscles.

- Avoid opening the mouth too wide — this helps to protect the joints and further prevents them from locking open.

- Yawn against pressure.

- Try to eat small bites.

- Apply cold for 5-10 minutes for severe pain due to new injuries (less than 72 hours).

- Apply moist heat for 20 minutes against an aching muscle for mild to moderate pain to increase circulation and muscle relaxation, which promotes healing.

- Massage the jaw and the temple muscles. This process stimulates proper circulation of blood, relaxes muscles and decrease soreness.

- Yoga and meditation help to relieve the body and reduce stress.

- Maintain good posture — avoid a forward head posture that may enhance both jaw and muscle activity and soreness.

- Use of over-the-counter medications — the medications are more helpful to prevent pain and inflammation, e.g., take two aspirin or ibuprofen four times daily, according to directions on the label.

- Sleep on one side. Support both neck and shoulders with a pillow with a soft support along the face and the jaw. You can also sleep with your back of the neck supported.

## Treatment options

TMJ is generally a self-limiting disorder since the pain and clicking of the syndrome infrequently become more serious. Most symptoms of TMJ syndrome usually improve without medical treatment or within three to six months of non-surgical treatment. However, in some cases, treatment is required if:

- Patient has a medical history of inflammatory joint disease.

- Symptoms do not improve after six months.

- There is progressive difficulty in opening the mouth.

- There is an inability to eat a normal diet.

- There is recurrent dislocation of the temporomandibular joint.

### Primary Option

Ibuprofen: 400 mg orally three times daily when required for 14 days, maximum 3200 mg/day

Naproxen: 250-500 mg orally twice daily when required for 14 days, maximum 1250 mg/day

Diclofenac sodium: 50-100 mg orally twice daily when required for 14 days, maximum 150 mg/day

Patients with osteoarthritis and persistent pain after two weeks of joint rest are required to take non-steroidal anti-inflammatory drugs (NSAIDs) since it helps to relieve pain and inflammation. However, this drug inhibits platelet aggregation and cause gastric irritation if used for a longer time. It also increases the risk of hepatotoxicity and nephrotoxicity. Moreover, dentists should be cautious when prescribing this drug to patients with bleeding disorders or with kidney or liver disorders.

Myofascial pain does not respond to NSAIDs because inflammation is not the cause of chronic muscle pain in the oro-facial region. Other drugs like diazepam are effective in treating pain due to its muscle-relaxant effects. If needed, a 10-day course of treatment can be started following a two-week trial of joint rest. Caution should be used in prescribing diazepam, as drowsiness and dependence can occur. NSAIDs are effective in treating the symptoms of internal systemic derangement/dysfunction and osteoarthritic subtypes of TMJ syndrome.

## Conservative treatment

Conservative treatment of TMJ syndrome can be justified by two reasons. First, the condition is self-remitting in approximately three-quarters of all TMJ cases and progress to a large degree occurs within three months of initiation (Thomson et.al., 2013)[12]. The second factor encouraging a conservative approach is the occurrence of the disorder. Bradley (1987)[13] stated that at least one of the main symptoms of TMJ, clicking, locking, or pain in the TMJ, had been experienced by approximately one-fifth of the general population by the age of 30 years. TMJ conservative treatments include:

## Botox (Botulinum Toxin A)

Using Botox injections as TMJ treatment provides significant and immediate relief in some patients and has shown positive results in recent years. Individuals who possess notable trigger points with contracted muscles or who experience muscles spasms with headaches are perfect candidates for injection of botulinum toxin A.

The industrial name of botulinum toxin type A is Botox. It is produced from Clostridium botulinum, a strain of the bacterium. Injection of Botox into the muscles leads to blockage of the signals sent from the brain, which results in muscle contraction. Furthermore, Botox disarms the muscular target, thus blocking the panic signal transmission throughout the body and forcing the body to believe that no pain is felt. Botox is quite useful in relaxing the muscle for three to six months, after which the muscles spontaneously contract on their own without spasms or pain.

### Procedure

Injections of Botox are conducted on an outpatient basis in many clinics, after which the patient is allowed to leave when the treatment is successfully completed. The procedure begins with location of the trigger points, which are marked with a pen. The identified area is then sterilized with an antiseptic spray called chlorhexidine. The injection of the local anesthetic follows through a small cosmetic needle.

Botox is injected using three different methods. Typically, the use of small cosmetic needles is the first option; however, if the trigger points prove to be hard to access, a Stimuplex nerve stimulator or ultrasound guidance is sometimes used. The Botox dosage should be close to 100 units; however, this can range up to 200 units, depending on the area affected.

## Outcome

One of the merits of using Botox is that there is little or no recovery time, since most patients resume their normal life immediately after treatment. Results usually last for 3-6 months and the process can be repeated.

## Dry needling

TMJ dysfunction can cause an assortment of problems, including pain in many areas, such as the joint, facial muscles, and the ear, as well as headaches, loss of jaw range of motion, tinnitus, and many others. Pain in the muscles is often caused by spasms. Many of us are familiar with TMJ from the popping sound we hear in our jaws as we chew.

Dry needling is used to relax contracted muscles, improve blood and lymphatic circulation, and stimulate the stretch reflex in muscles. While needles are used in this treatment, dry needling must not be confused with acupuncture. The way it works is that a dry needle is inserted into areas of the muscles, known as trigger points. Certain trigger points are associated with pain in certain parts of the body. The needle in the trigger point causes a contracted muscle to twitch, which disrupts the neurological feedback loop that keeps the muscle in the contracted state. This twitch causes the muscle spasm to release, leading to restoration of the normal neuromuscular function.

## Myofunctional therapy

Orofacial myofunctional therapy (OMT) is used to treat various oral myofunctional disorders. The process involves a series of exercises used to re-pattern and optimize oral and facial functions. OMT is a neuromuscular re-education of the muscles involved in swallowing, chewing, and mandibular posture using specific exercises targeting the muscle groups. OMT uses behavior modification by introducing and habituating static and dynamic coordinated patterns that promote stable and correct oral postures. Oral myofunctional disorders exert pressures against oral structures that lead to the disruption of normal muscle patterns, thus negatively impacting growth and development of head and neck. Common oral myofunctional disorders include damaging oral habits (thumb sucking, nail biting), lack of proper lip seal when the jaw is at rest, chronic mouth breathing, forward tongue and head posture, increased vertical freeway space, aberrant swallowing patterns (tongue thrusts) and tongue-ties. OMDs have been associated with various disorders, including sleep disordered breathing/sleep apnea, craniomandibular malalignment and cranial distortions, malocclusions and altered dental development, periodontal disease, speech problems, gastroesophageal reflux disease, bruxism, orthodontic relapse, and TMJ.

### The treatment is divided into four phases

1. Pre-treatment (elimination of noxious oral habits)

2. Intensive phase (weekly appointments for eight weeks), during which time the therapist and patient work on

muscle activation, lips together at rest, palatal tongue rest position, chewing and swallowing of food and liquids, coordinating and patterning orofacial muscles to attain proper function. This reinforces any habit elimination.

3. Generalization Phase (appointments are once every 2-3 weeks for approximately 2-4 months). Exercises are tailored to maintain a new pattern of swallowing, integrate awareness into activities day and night regarding oral rest posture, and habits are observed.

4. Habituation Phase (therapist monitors patient with monthly evaluations and exercises until treatment program is complete, approximately one year). Follow-up is scheduled as needed.

## Stem cell therapy

Stem cell therapy is a field of study in the treatment of temporomandibular joint disorders. In brief, a TMJ disorder is the result of damage to the ligaments or elements of the TMJ. This joint is essential to chewing and speaking. Such a disorder can result in a great deal of pain in and around the jaw, face, ears, and even the neck and shoulders. People with this condition may experience difficulty chewing and opening their mouths wide, and a popping or grating sound may accompany the movement of the jaw.

Up until recently, this type of disorder was considered by many to be extremely difficult to treat. Fortunately, stem cell therapy has become a serious contender as a potential long-term solution.

Procedures for this type of treatment have varied among specialists. Some practitioners use the patient's own stem cells to treat the TMJ. These cells are collected with a minimally invasive procedure, similar to liposuction, together with the fat in which the cells are found. The cells are then separated from the fat within 90 minutes, and the stem cells are injected into the TMJ using a tiny needle. More stem cells are given intravenously to reach the joint and other affected areas via the bloodstream.

Though stem therapy is still under research, we are optimistic because stem cells have so far proven to be very promising in regenerating cartilage in TMJs. This opens the possibility for a long-term cure for sufferers from temporomandibular joint disorders.

Stem cell treatment for TMJ is still a new approach and must be considered experimental at this time, in spite of the almost proven benefit. However, in view of the extremely low risk of the procedure, we are very optimistic that this method will become one of the standard choices of management for people suffering from TMJ disorder.

## Transcutaneous electrical nerve stimulation

Transcutaneous electrical nerve stimulation (TENS) therapy is fundamentally the application of a device to administer a pulsed electrical current of low voltage. TENS produces a two-phase wave of asymmetric or symmetric current, balanced as a negative square semi-wave and a positive peak. Upon application to the skin surface by electrodes, its aim is to loosen up agitated muscles and encourage pain alleviation.

TENS produces different pulse frequencies that vary in intensity as well as duration. It is classified into two categories, a high frequency of 50Hz and above/low frequency of 10Hz. TENS used in dentistry mixes high- and low-frequency currents. High-frequency pulses of about 50 to 150 Hz have low intensity, and they seem to be basically central, even though more studies are contentious about its action on chronic pain. The use of low frequency has fundamentally marginal success for muscle relaxation. During the procedure, the intensity should be adjusted to avoid muscle contractions, obtain hypoesthesia (decreased sensation) around the treated region and paresthesia (loss of sensation) of the region being treated by regulating the machine in accordance with the patient's sensitivity. Appropriate intensities should vary from 10-30 milliamps since they produce few fasciculations. Pulse time values should vary between 40 and 75 microseconds.

TENS is used in dentistry controls chronic pain in preferred areas and relaxes masticatory muscles. Experimental studies have revealed that, at rest, muscles of TMD patients possess higher myoelectric action of jaw elevator muscles than those in control groups, projected in the anterior segment of the temporal muscle. Application of TENS has facilitated pain relief with instantaneous myoelectric activity in the anterior segment of the muscles. In addition, an increase in the electromyographic amplitude of jaw elevator muscles is most likely due to sensory-motor connections of the craniofacial segment that might adjust action potential generation and the activity of myoelectric amplitude.

TENS impacts, conversely, are built on diverse speculative bases, such as the idea that stimulating motor nerves directly leads masticatory muscles to perform rhythmic contractions. The recurring movement of skeletal muscles, as well as mild rhythmic movement, hastens the flow of local blood, thus reducing noxious metabolites that have built up in the tissues and interstitial edema. This process reduces the pain, thus increasing energetic accessibility of phosphate radicals, muscle hypoxia reduction, and fatigue in masticatory muscles (Christensen et.al., 1991)[20]. TENS is a comparatively cost-effective and non-invasive and is a safe healing modality that might be used to cure numerous painful situations. TENS electrodes are made of silicone gel that is applied between the device and the body skin.

Many studies have revealed the efficiency of using TENS to treat TMD in combination with other therapies to improve stomatognathic system functionality. Regarding the same issue, other studies (Tanne et. al., 2002)[21] reported that patients with TMD have hyperactivity in the masticatory muscles while the jaw is resting and this causes ischemia, fatigue in the muscles, functional pain, and disorders.

TENS has the efficacy to relieve different types of pain. Due to specific masticatory system characteristics, TENS for pain and temporomandibular disorder should also be used against those unique qualities. In this sense, further controlled studies with homogeneous samples of TMD patients are needed to confirm the beneficial aspects of this therapy to control craniofacial pain.

## Diathermy, infrared, and ultrasound treatment

Ultrasonic therapy or ultrasonic diathermy devices incorporated into physical therapy equipment produce high-frequency sound waves that travel deep into tissue and create gentle therapeutic heat. Ultrasonic diathermy is intended to generate deep heat within body tissues for the treatment of selected medical conditions such as pain, muscle spasms, and joint contractures, but not for the treatment of malignancies.

The sound waves are transmitted through a round-headed wand that the therapist applies to the skin with gentle, circular movements. A hypo-allergenic gel aids in the transmission of the ultrasonic energy and prevents overheating at the surface of the applicator. Treatments usually last between five and ten minutes. Ultrasonic therapy does not hurt (there may be a bit of a tingling sensation and/or a sensation of warmth) if the therapist keeps the wand moving continuously. If, however, the wand is held in place for more than a few seconds, it can become uncomfortable at higher energies.

**Things to know**

While ultrasonic therapy can be used to treat the conditions described above, it is important to know that there are situations and areas of the body where it cannot be safely used. Patients should notify the practitioner administering the ultrasound if any of the following is applicable to you

☐ You have a cardiac pacemaker.

☐ You have a malignancy in the area to be treated.

☐ You have a healing fracture in the area to be treated.

☐ You are pregnant.

☐ You have an implanted medical device other than a pacemaker, such as implanted deep brain stimulation device.

Patients should also be aware that commercial ultrasonic diathermy devices may exist that have not been formally evaluated by FDA. Typically, these devices will claim to treat a range of diseases and disorders and are purported to have other uses that are not covered in the description above (for example, to reduce wrinkles on the face). It is always best to avoid such practice and get consultation from an approved authority.

## Relaxation therapy

Relaxation therapy is a common component of the treatment for TMJ disorder since stress leads to jaw-clenching and teeth-grinding. This therapy's approach may include neck and shoulder physical therapy to relax these muscles.

People with TMJ may suffer from sleep apnea or heavy snoring, which aggravates TMJ disorder. Other treatments include hydrotheraphy, hypnosis/relaxation therapy, dental restoration, intra-articular injection of hyaluronic acid, etc.

## Surgical interventions

Replacement of the temporomandibular joint with an artificial implant should only be considered as a last resort. When used in patients who have had multiple prior jaw surgeries, it may improve function, but studies have shown that it generally does not significantly reduce pain. Before undergoing such surgery on the jaw joint, it is extremely important to get other independent opinions and to fully understand the potential benefits and significant risks of the procedure under consideration.

TMJ surgery may be considered medically necessary in cases where there is conclusive evidence that severe pain or functional disability is produced by an intra-capsular condition, confirmed by magnetic resonance imaging (MRI), computed tomography or other imaging, that has not responded to non-surgical management, and surgery is considered to be the only remaining option.

Non-surgical management includes three or more months of the following, where appropriate:

- professional physical therapy,

- pharmacological therapy,

- behavioral therapy (such as cognitive behavioral therapy or relaxation therapy),

- manipulation (for reduction of dislocation or fracture of the TMJ), and

- reversible intra-oral appliances (unless the patient is unable to open the mouth wide enough).

In certain cases (e.g., bony ankylosis and failed TMJ total joint prosthetic implants) that require immediate surgical intervention, surgery may be considered medically necessary without prior non-surgical management.

**Note:** All requests for surgery must include documentation that all medically appropriate non-surgical therapies listed above have been exhausted. Surgical methods are only applied when:

- ☐ There is identifiable pathology amenable to surgical intervention.

- ☐ There is a resultant loss of mechanical function.

- ☐ There is pain related to joint pathology.

- ☐ Any of the above has failed to respond to non-interventional treatment and there is, as a result, persistent loss of normal mandibular function that is negatively affecting the patient's wellbeing in a persistent and unremitting manner.

☐ There has been a thorough explanation of the relative pros and cons of a specific intervention, a review of the potential benefits, risks, and complications.

A surgical assessment (workup) will include:

☐ A complete review of the nature of the TMD and all treatment attempts to date.

☐ Radiographic assessment, including any or all of the following: dental panoramic radiographs, CT scan, MRI or bone scan.

☐ A thorough medical assessment, including medical risk factors that may affect the surgical outcome.

The following TMJ articular disorders are manageable with surgical intervention:

☐ Internal derangements (disc displacement disorders)

☐ Non-inflammatory (non-infective degenerative disorders; post-traumatic degeneration)

☐ Inflammatory disease (osteomyelitis, synovitis, lupus, psoriasis, rheumatoid arthritis)

☐ Neoplasia

☐ Ankylosis

The following is a review of the surgical procedures that can be employed in the management of TMJ.

# Condylectomy

Condylectomy is one of the medical procedures used to treat TMJ disorders (also known simply as TMD). This is a surgical procedure used in cases that involve an organic disease of the joint. It works by totally removing the condyle.

The TMJ is a condylar joint at the main joint of the jaw. It connects the mandible and the temporal bone, hence its name. It is made up of mandibular condyles, the articular surface of the temporal bone, an articular disc, a lateral pterygoid, a capsule, and ligaments. The TMJ's main function is to allow jaw movement. As such, it plays a key role in eating and speaking.

When any of the structures of the TMJ is displaced or damaged for any reason, TMJ disorders develop. These disorders can be dealt with through surgical procedures such as condylectomy.

Condylectomy is beneficial for patients who suffer from temporomandibular joint disorders. These include:

☐ Degenerative joint disease (DJD), or diseases that are characterized by inflamed joints and tissues surrounding the jaw.

☐ Internal derangement, such as disc displacement with reduction.

☐ Displaced condyle fractures or when the condyle bone becomes fractured.

☐ Recurrent luxations or recurrent dislocations.

☐ Ankylosis, or the abnormal immobility of a joint resulting from fibrosis or bone union; it can be caused by disease, injury, or surgery.

☐ Temporal arteritis, or inflammation of the blood vessels that supply blood to the temporal area (head and neck).

- Myofascial pain disorder, a painful condition of the TMJ caused by muscle tension and spasms.

However, condylectomy is more effective in patients who suffer from organic TMJ disorders or those that are stress-related. These disorders typically cause symptoms, such as:

- Clicking or popping noise when the patient chews or moves his jaws
- Muscle pain around the jaw
- Pain around the ear that spreads to the cheeks and temples
- Headache or migraine
- Tight or stuck jaw
- Difficulty opening the mouth
- Earache
- Blocked sensation in the jaw
- Pain in the neck
- Backache
- Sleep disturbances
- Facial asymmetry

## How is the procedure performed?

A condylectomy, which can be either low or high, removes the condyle completely. A high condylectomy is a modified version of the procedure in which the bone of the condyle head is simply recontoured to remove the diseased or damaged part. This is effective in removing any bone irregularities or impingement in the temporomandibular joint. The procedure is commonly performed on the lateral part of the joint.

The procedure usually takes 60 to 90 minutes. After the surgery, the patient is usually advised to stay in the hospital for 24 hours. Condylectomy is sometimes combined with other procedures, such as a caudal mandibulectomy. This is most effective on patients who have periarticular neoplasia or ankylosis. It can also be performed in conjunction with orthognathic surgery. Condylectomies are also usually followed by a reconstruction procedure.

## Possible risks and complications

The complication rate of condylectomy procedures for the treatment of TMJ disorders is very low. Most patients undergo the procedure without any complication. In a study involving 14 patients, none of them had any pain during the follow-up visit.

A condylectomy is therefore considered a safe procedure. There are only a few potential complications and they are mostly related to the temporal branch of the facial nerve. These include:

☐ Scarring, which is usually insignificant and does not cause major esthetic problems for most patients.

☐ TMJ noises, which occurred in three patients (or 21.4% of the participants in the study).

☐ Compromised facial nerve function.

☐ Facial nerve injury.

☐ Limited jaw movement.

☐ Decrease in the vertical dimension of the surgical site, resulting in an open bite.

# Arthrocentesis

Arthrocentesis with insufflation, lysis, and lavage is considered medically necessary when imaging and a clinical examination reveal an anchored disc phenomenon, anterior disc displacement without reduction and without effusion, osteoarthritis without fibrosis or loose bone particles, open lock, or hemarthrosis (blood in the joint space).

Arthrocentesis for TMJ internal derangement is the insertion of two separate single needle portals or a single double needle portal for the input and output of fluids. The process includes insufflation of the joint space, lavage, manipulation of the mandible to achieve lysis of adhesions, and the elective infusion of steroids.

## Therapeutic arthroscopy

Therapeutic arthroscopy is considered medically necessary when MRI or other imaging confirms the presence of adhesions, fibrosis, degenerative joint disease, or internal derangement of the disc that requires internal modification.

Open surgical procedures including, but not limited to, meniscus or disc repositioning or plication, disc repair, and disc removal with or without replacement are considered medically necessary when TMJ dysfunction is the result of congenital anomalies, trauma, or disease in patients for whom non-surgical management has failed.

## Arthroplasty

Arthroplasty or arthrotomy is an umbrella word that refers to a group of TMJ surgical procedures approached with an incision directly into the joint itself. This procedure is more useful to patients with progressive debilitating internal derangement refractory to the non-surgical and minimally invasive techniques. The surgical procedures include:

- ☐ Disk repair.

- ☐ Diskectomy with or without replacement.

- ☐ Articular surface recontouring (condylectomy and eminectomy or eminoplasty). Arthroplasty or arthrotomy is considered medically necessary when MRI or other imaging confirms the presence of any of the following:

  - o Osteoarthritis or osteoarthrosis.

  - o Severe disc displacement associated with degenerative changes or perforation.

  - o Severe scarring that is often the result of an old injury or prior procedure.

Surgical treatments are controversial and should be avoided, if possible. There have been no long-term clinical trials to study the safety and effectiveness of surgical treatments for TMD, nor are there criteria to identify people who would most likely benefit from surgery. Failure to respond to conservative treatments, for example, does not automatically signify that more aggressive treatments, such as surgery, are necessary. If you have had prior joint surgery, remember that another surgical procedure is not always the answer to the problem.

## Prognosis and complications

The prognosis for TMJ syndrome is generally good. There are numerous causes for TMJ syndrome and the outlook depends on the cause, if known. Most people can manage the discomfort with self-care and home remedies. Furthermore, complications of long-term TMJ syndrome include chronic face pain or chronic headaches. In severe situations, where the pain is chronic or associated with other inflammatory disorders, long-term treatment may be necessary.

TMJ syndrome is a self-limiting disorder since the signs and symptoms decrease with age. With time, clicking in the TMJ decreases, so most patients will likely improve with or without treatment. Treatment of TMJ syndrome is not curative, but palliative; 80% of patients will be successfully managed with palliative treatment.

## Treatment of disability and complications

Individuals who have TMJ can usually handle the symptoms through self-care, such as:

- avoiding chewing hard foods,

- icing the jaw, or

- taking over-the-counter medications for pain.

However, if the TMJ is severe enough, it can affect other parts of the body and can even lead to disability. Complications might include chronic facial pain, and wearing, cracking, or misalignment of the teeth (malocclusion).

Patients with refractory pain or disability, such as with osteoarthritis or internal derangement, should undergo surgery. Surgical procedures include arthrocentesis, condylotomy, and even total TMJ replacement. However, it must always be remembered that surgery is reserved for patients who have moderate to severe pain, have notable pathology, and are disabled by their condition.

## Follow-ups/evaluations

✦ Patients on analgesics or with splints should be followed up at four-week intervals.

✦ Every patient must be carefully instructed and prescribed the appropriate medication and measures.

✦ Patients being treated with occlusal splints/night guards should be instructed to follow up with a dentist one week after receiving the appliance. The splint should be checked for appropriate fitting and comfort.

## Using 'multidisciplinary approach' — how and why?

A multidisciplinary form of approach in the treatment of TMJ disorder works toward a better outcome to capture the richness of experience in the lives of patients and to boost patients' confidence, along with achieving normal form, function, and stability of the joint. This approach has shown a lot of improvement: Many patients have experienced positive results, not only in terms of aesthetics and function but also profoundly positive influences on psychological development, self-esteem, and self-confidence.

TMJ disorder impacts facial and head features differently, resulting in differences in both appearance and speech. Management of the psychosocial adjustment of a patient with poor facial appearance has moved from the development of adaptation toward the optimum results deserved by the patient through a team approach. Many studies have displayed significant improvement by employing treatment through a phase-wise multidisciplinary approach.

A multidisciplinary approach involves a combination of various processes to effectively manage TMJ. This combination is carried out in a stepwise manner. The following breakdown explains this approach more elaborately.

## Surgery

The initial surgery is conducted under general anesthesia. Gap arthroplasty is then conducted through the preauricular approach. After exposing and identifying the site of the disorder, aggressive excision of the fibrous and/or bony mass is carried out with round bur and chisel until the mandibular movement is achieved. Next, the glenoid fossa is recontoured as necessary (as per gap opening). For total TMJ reconstruction, after resection, a costochondral graft is put in place in order to reconstruct the TMJ.

The surgery can be slightly modified and improvised from patient to patient, but the end goal remains the same: to achieve success in curing the patient.

## Physiotherapy

Physiotherapy is the second stage after surgery. Extensive physiotherapy usually plays a crucial role in restoring normal TMJ function. Physiotherapy entails exercising the masticatory muscles, lips, and tongue to increase the mobility of the mandible. Moreover, chewing on a rubber tube is recommended to stimulate normal mastication. Physiotherapy also employs the aggressive use of continuous passive movement and tongue blades.

## Restorative and oral prophylactic care

Restoration of carious teeth and oral prophylactic measures are necessary once the goal of the mouth opening to its maximum is achieved by the patient. Furthermore, the patients should be trained on how to perform daily prophylactic oral hygiene measures.

## Fixed orthodontic mechanotherapy

Fixed orthodontic mechanotherapy, with all first pre-molars extracted to resolve bimaxillary protrusion, is initiated for the alignment and establishment of occlusion, using a fix-bonded orthodontic appliance. After alignment and leveling are completed within two and half months, all first pre-molars are extracted and space closure is done with maximum conservation of posterior anchorage. After 14 months of treatment, the patient has a good dental relationship, with the upper and lower anterior teeth retracted and positioned upright into near-normal positions over the basal bone. Space closure is completed without the development of an anterior open bite or deep overbite. With the retraction of the lips, the patient's profile and smile are improved. Once the result is achieved, the fixed appliance and retainers are de-bonded.

## Genioplasty

Six months after completion of orthodontic treatment, sliding advancement genioplasty is performed. The process is rather simple and involves conducting chin advancement and alignment procedure by fixation with a titanium plate.

## Speech and functional therapy

Concern regarding speech is paramount and is thought to be equally important as appearance in contributing to low self-esteem in patients. Unusual speech due to jaw thrusting is a major problem faced by many patients. Therefore, a thorough evaluation for the speech therapy is required to determine problems, such as a mixed type of articulation disorder, i.e., omission, substitution, and distortion types. Whenever such disorders are observed, patients are prepared for speech therapy, and major training commences once they achieve sufficient jaw movements after TMJ surgery. Speech and functional therapy improve articulation defects after joint surgery and orthodontic dentoalveolar corrections. Moreover, speech and functional therapy completely eliminate lisping of sound after orthodontic corrections.

## Psychological counseling

Lastly, psychometric tests are used to identify adversity in the experience of TMJ disorder, mostly due to poor facial appearance. Psychological counseling evaluates the thoughts and feelings about facial disfigurement in the pre- and post-treatment stages using standardized psychometric questionnaires that have been developed, validated, and used by social scientists and psychologists.

After careful evaluation, counseling is done and certain sessions are held with the patient where s/he is taught how to overcome psychological issues and depression that generally comes with this problem.

## Concurrent Therapies

## Antidepressants

Antidepressants, such as tricyclic antidepressants and serotonin-reuptake inhibitors, help relieve pain and improve mood in patients with TMJ.

## Hyaluronic acid

Several studies found that intra-articular injections of hyaluronic acid in dysfunctional temporomandibular joints had favorable outcomes. Intra-articular injection of HA is recommended in dysfunction of the TMJ; however, further studies are required to establish therapeutic impacts and identification of the dosage regimen.

## Acupuncture

Several studies have evaluated the effectiveness of acupuncture in the treatment of TMJ syndrome. Acupuncture has been found to relieve TMJ pain in some randomized studies, but more trials are necessary. Pain relief is usually short term. Acupuncture helps relieve pain by releasing endogenous opioids along with serotonin and norepinephrine in the dorsal horn of the spinal cord. However, there are specific acupoints that should be used for TMJ syndrome. Acupuncture treatment can be given weekly for a total of six treatments and can be used as an adjunct to more traditional TMJ syndrome treatment.

## Low-level laser therapy

Low-level laser therapy has been used to treat temporomandibular disorders with varied and controversial outcomes. Further study is needed in this regard, too.

# Chapter 4: Self-care and home cure

This section deals with helping you find hope with your chronic temporomandibular joint condition. We will learn easy and effective life hacks and tips to make your life better right in the comfort of your home.

Below are some TMJ exercises that not only relieve pain but also improve the function of the joint:

### Exercise #01

This entails opening the mouth as wide as you can without feeling any pain. Move the jaw slowly while holding the mouth open; hold it on the right for 10 seconds. Return it to the center, then move the jaw steadily to the left and grasp it for another 10 seconds. Return the jaw to middle and then close the mouth. The procedure is repeated for the next 4 to 5 minutes.

### Exercise #02

This workout involves the use of the index finger. On the right side, locate the jaw hinge and softly massage it with a downward movement of the finger. The same procedure is applied on the left side using the left index finger.

### Exercise #03

Open the mouth wide without feeling any pain. While keeping the mouth wide open, shift the tongue tip upwards to contact the uppermost part of the mouth. Holding the tongue in the same position, move the tip of the tongue to the backward position, i.e., toward the tonsils, then hold it for the next 5 seconds. Stick the tongue out and stretch it out as far as possible for 5 seconds. Repeat this procedure 5 to 10 times.

## Exercise #04

Sitting in an upright position, shift the chin up and down for one minute. Stop momentarily, and then change the chin movement to sideways positions for another minute. Repeat the same exercise twice. Avoid stretching too hard and spraining the neck.

## Exercise #05

While standing in front of a mirror, hold the chin and support it using both hands, after which open the jaws wide and stretch the tip of the tongue to touch the roof of the mouth. Holding the tip of the tongue in the same position, move the jaws slowly up and down as you apply slight resistance with the hands every time the jaws open. The process is done for one minute in every session and should be repeated thrice a day.

## Exercise #06

Without hurting the mouth, yawn as wide as the mouth can stretch. Repeat yawning but, this time, do it twice more while opening the mouth in halfway wide position. Repeat the same procedure twice.

## Relaxation exercises

Psychological factors, such as stress, are the major cause of TMJ. Exercises that ease and relax the central nervous system and the spinal cord are helpful home remedies for TMJ disorders. Below is a wonderful spine exercise to help you relax.

Sit in an upright position and turn the head forward so that the chin touches the chest. Interlock the fingers of both hands and put them behind the head. Resist the backward movement by using the hands while pushing the head back. Avoid pushing the head with force. The same procedure is supposed to be repeated 3-5 twice a day so as to ease the spinal cord.

While sitting in a vertical position, open the mouth to a relaxed position. Bend the head back so that the forehead points up to the sky. Inhale deeply and gradually exhale. Resume the initial position and repeat the process.

This is a deep breathing exercise: While lying on your back, place the left hand on the stomach and rest the right hand on the chest. Relax for some few minutes, after which inhale deeply, allow the air to pass through the trachea to the stomach. Slowly release the air. Repeat this procedure 10-20 minutes per exercise.

Other simple relaxation exercise includes walking, jogging, playing tennis, and cycling, which facilitate blood pumping. Yoga exercises and meditation are also useful to stimulate relaxation. Habitual exercising methods are also significant to reduce stress.

## Eating habits

### Hydration of the body

Disorders such as muscle cramps of the neck, mandibular joints, and shoulders are caused by lack of efficient water in the body. The body should be properly hydrated because dehydration causes TMJ-related disorders. You should increase daily water intake; the minimum intake should be eight glasses (150 ounces) a day. You should also distribute intake evenly throughout the day. Intake of excess water within a short period of time is not advised since it can cause hyper-hydration. Therefore, drinking two glasses of water every two hours is recommended.

## Role of nutrition

Lack of essential minerals increases TMJ pain. Studies have shown that, out of 280 TMJ patients, 249 lack essential minerals, such as calcium and magnesium. On the other hand, a study carried out by the International Dentist Association using 50 TMJ patients showed that eating food with additional magnesium and calcium supplements eased TMJ symptoms by 70%.

Calcium strengthens the bones while magnesium is useful for alleviating pain in the muscles. Every normal person requires magnesium intake of about 310mg, which is not equally supplemented in the diet. Some of the notable symptoms include muscle spasms. Moreover, magnesium helps in calcium metabolism in the body, hence preventing TMJ disorders such as osteoporosis.

**List of foods rich in magnesium:**

Oats, molasses, cashew nuts, sunflower, Brazilian nuts, corn, sesame butter, sunflower seeds, wheat and black-eyed peas.

**List of foods rich in calcium:**

A normal person requires a daily intake of 10 grams of calcium. Foods rich in calcium are unpolished rice, banana, spinach, coconut, milk, sesame, green peas, and cabbage. Change the diet by removing junk foods and replacing them with nuts, vegetables, grains, and fresh fruits to alleviate TMJ symptoms and pain.

# Supplements

### Vitamin B-complex

Lack of Vitamin B is also referred as induced stress, which results in TMJ pain. To curb the deficiency, average adults are advised to take Vitamin B-complex capsules for 15 days.

### Glucosamine sulfate

This mineral builds and repairs cartilage in our body; it also relieves pain and stiffness and helps to prevent swelling in the joints due to diseases such as TMJ, osteoarthritis, rheumatism, and other disorders. It is also effective if TMJ has cartilage deterioration. Some of the natural sources of glucosamine sulfate are Gingko Biloba, spinach, and glucosamine.

## Lifestyle modification ideas

### Sitting position

Poor sitting position is the main cause of TMJ pain. Individuals should make a habit of sitting in an upright position. If, for an example, your job entails sitting in the office for a longer time, make sure the chair has good lumbar support. Schedule some breaks to stretch and relax the spinal cord.

### Hot massage

For the proper relief of TMJ pain, use a heating pad to massage the jaw, shoulders, and the neck. Hot massage is regarded as a useful muscle relaxant. A hot bath can equally help in this regard.

### Cold packs

Application of cold packs to the jaw and around the neck is useful for alleviating TMJ pains and related symptoms. To apply a cold pack, the plastic zipper bag should be filled with ice and covered with a cloth. Put the cloth on the affected neck and jaw for as long as you feel comfortable. Alternatively, a cold massage is also very effective in providing relief from TMJ pain.

### Body massage

Massaging the body with sandalwood, tea tree, juniper, bergamot, or oil helps to improve the circulation, thus relieving TMJ symptoms.

## NOTE

Most antibiotic pills and contraceptives reduce human immunity and increase strain within the muscles, which aggravates TMJ disorders. Discussion of all pills is paramount before use to prevent TMJ-related issues.

## Herbal options

In many cases of TMJ, it has been found that doctors keep looking for local causes of pain and fail to diagnose the exact cause. The result? The patient often fails to respond to treatment, so the frustration and anxiety increase.

For an effective cure, it is important to correctly diagnose the cause. Once diagnosed, proper treatment can provide psychological and physical relief. Pain caused by muscular contraction can be temporarily relieved with medication, exercises, or psychological therapy. But the root cause of disease (e.g., malocclusion dislocation) still persists.

Alternatively, doctors prescribe surgery of blood vessels in the brain to realign temporomandibular joints in an optimal position. This neuromuscular and dental surgery mostly provides relief from chronic pain. However, surgery is expensive and not without post-surgical complications. Some patients may consult a chiropractor or other doctors to treat other allied symptoms of TMJ.

Certain herbs are effective in the treatment of TMJ disorders. Common herbs used to alleviate TMJ include:

- **Magnesia Phosphorica:** Antispasmodic that relieves stiff muscles.

- **Methylsulfonylmethane:** this herb decreases inflammation and muscular spasm.

- **Rhus Toxicodendron:** it loosens stiff jaw.

- **Valerian Officinalis:** relaxes tension in the muscles.

- **Kava:** eases the nervous system.

- **Kali Phosphorica**: lessens nerve pain,

A portion of the herbs can be massaged into the jaws to give relief from TMJ-related pain. Other herbs that are useful in the treatment of TMJ are:

## Herbs for TMJ relief

**Ginger, *i.e., Zingiber officinale***

Damp herb is recommended for TMJ patients. Sporadic application of five ginger doses every five minutes can help relieve the pain in ears and sinus, while 5-15 drops of neti pot with tincture is wonderful for quick rinsing.

## Wild Ginger, *i.e., Asarum canadense*

Wild ginger is quite useful when the sinuses are dry and cracked. Moreover, wild ginger warms the body and produces body sweat and lubrication. Ginger produces more heat and is therefore not suitable. Wild ginger in combination with other herbs, such as plantain, dandelion, and ragweed flowers forms a perfect neti pot tincture that soothes the sinuses, thus helping to relieve TMJ pains and painful ears when other things do not work.

## Mullein, i.e., *Verbascum thapsus*

Mullein is an herb used in the treatment of the TMJ since it aids relief from the symptoms. For proper management of the pain associated with TMJ, use the first leaf or the yellow blossoms. Putting a few drops of the mullein blossom oil in the ear as you lie on the side helps a lot. Mullein blossom oil offers relief, especially when the oil goes deep into the Eustachian tubes. This oil helps a lot, especially after steam bathing or showering, since the sinuses are opened and the muscles are relaxed to facilitate the movement of the oil to the affected place.

## Herbs to reduce anxiety, stress, and tension

The principal medical fact underlying TMJ disorders is that psychological stress, anxiety, and tension are the main causes of the disorder. Therefore, incorporating sedatives and calming herbs are absolutely paramount to ease TMJ pain.

## Blue vervain, i.e., *Verbena hastata*

This herb is helpful for alleviating TMJ pain in many ways. It is used to relieve tension and anxiety problems. The tincture can be extracted from the flower, leaves, and roots. Daily doses of the tincture should be one dropper, up to three times a day to relieve the muscle tension in the jaw that results from the clenched bite. This tincture also helps to relieve the headaches, muscular pain, and pain in both sinuses that are associated with TMJ.

**Agrimony, i.e., *Agrimonia eupatoria***

This herb is the most important in releasing the muscle tension of the jaw that TMJ has stemmed from. It helps to ease the tension that can aggravate the inflammation of various sinuses and very stiff jaw joint.

## Musculoskeletal Herbs

Temporomandibular joint disorder erupts from tension and other aspects, such as psychological stress. Moreover, the pain normally manifests itself in the muscles. Therefore, if an individual is suffering from TMJ as the result of an injury, he/she requires a proper treatment with herbs because sedative drugs won't help him/her sufficiently or for the long term.

Despite linking TMJ with jaw problems, this disorder usually extends to the shoulders, neck, and muscles. Back, neck, or spinal injury aggravates TMJ pain, since the muscle affected pulls down the other, which finally stretches the jaw muscles, making it tight and tense. The stretching causes tightness of the jaw joint, which finally pops out. Such tightness contributes to the jaw joint eventually popping out of place. Some of the useful herbs include:

**Solomon's seal, i.e., *Polygonatum spp.***

This herb is more useful for relieving the joints and the muscles. It is used to lubricate the joints, thus reducing the pain by lessening the friction.Solomon's seal also helps the muscles to attain the correct amount of tightness and looseness by balancing out this factor. Moreover, TMJ is part of the jaw muscle; hence, this herb might be effective to loosen muscles that are clinched too tightly. Application of the salve of the root into the TMJ is the most appropriate as compared to the internal tincture.

**Blue Vervain, i.e., *Verbena hastata***

This herb is effective to ease tension, besides helping with psychological stress. Blue vervain is quite effective in the treatment of back and shoulder pain and the disorders in TMJ. It is also effective in the treatment of muscular and tension jaw pain.

## Natural cures for TMJ

### Home remedies

Home remedies for TMJ are of vital importance in allaying and getting rid of the root cause. The natural home remedies mentioned below are very useful in relieving TMJ symptoms like muscular pain, headache, and anxiety. Some handy over-the-counter remedies for this disorder include:

- ☐ Magnesium (250 mg 2-3x daily) helps relax the muscles and nervous system.

- ☐ Calcium (500 mg 2x daily) works with magnesium to aid in muscle relaxation.

- ☐ Kava (70 mg 3x daily) helps reduce anxiety and relax the muscles.

- ☐ MSM (1000 mg 3x daily) is a natural anti-inflammatory and reduces muscle spasms.

- ☐ B-complex (50 mg 2x daily) helps relieve the effects of stress.

## Chiropractic care

When muscles in the cervical spine get tight, it can also affect the TMJ. Chiropractic can help reduce this tension, reduce stress and improve TMJ symptoms fast.

## Essential oils

The best essential oils to relieve TMJ are peppermint oil, frankincense oil, and lavender oil. Peppermint relieves pain, frankincense reduces inflammation, and lavender relaxes tense muscles. Mix 1 drop of each oil with 1/4 tsp of coconut oil and rub onto the area of pain.

## Natural cures

Some of the natural remedies that help alleviate TMJ symptoms, such as a headache, anxiety, and muscular pain include:

1. Exercises related to jaw movement.
2. Full body relaxation to alleviate stress.
3. Monitoring and changing the eating habits that exacerbate the TMJ disorder.

## Exercises related to jaw movement

There are several jaw-related exercises that can help in alleviating the TMJ disorder. A few of them are listed below.

Exercise Routine 1:

☐ Fully open your mouth to the maximum extent (you should open your mouth up to the limit where there is no pain and discomfort and try not to exceed it).

☐ After fully opening your mouth, gradually move your jaw toward the right and hold for at least 10 seconds

☐ Now return your jaw to the center position and start the same process for the left side. Hold for at least 10 seconds and then bring your jaw back to the middle.

☐ Close your mouth and let it relax. You should repeat this process five times daily.

Exercise routine 2:

Use the index finger of the right hand to trace the location of the jaw hinge on the right side of your face. Massage the hinge area, using a downward action with the finger. Repeat the same process for the left side of the face by using the index finger of the left hand.

Exercise routine 3:

Fully open the mouth to the maximum extent. Stick the tip of the tongue to reach the upper mouth, touching the roof of the upper mouth, and stretch the tongue toward the side of the tonsils. Hold to the maximum extent of the stretch for at least 5 seconds. Relax and then repeat the process again 5 to 10 times.

Exercise Routine 4:

Sit in a straight posture and perform an up-and-down movement with your chin for a minute. After that, perform side-to-side chin movement, again for a minute. Repeat the process (do the process in a relaxed manner to avoid injury).

## Full body relaxation to alleviate the stress

One of the major causes of the TMJ disorder is stressful living. Performing exercises that relax the nervous system and spinal cord prove to be efficient in gaining relief from the TMJ issues.

Some of the exercises that help alleviate the pain associated with TMJ disorder include:

Exercise Routine 1:

Sit in a straight posture and bend the head forward so that the chin touches the chest, then interlock the fingers and place them behind the head; push the head back and resist this movement using the hands placed at the back of the head. Repeat this process for at least three times but don't press the head very hard when following this routine.

Exercise Routine 2:

Sit in a straight posture, open the mouth and face the sky while bending the head in a backward direction so that the forehead points to the sky. Gulp a deep breath and resume the normal position.

Exercise Routine 3:

Lie down comfortably on the back and relax, keeping the right hand on the chest and the left hand on the stomach, and then take a deep breath. Concentrate on the breathing activity and do not think about anything else. Take heavy breaths at least 10 to 20 times in a single routine.

## Modifying your eating habits

A cracking sensation in the joints is a common complaint when chewing something, especially with TMJ disorder. The remedy is to avoid aggressive chewing and modify the daily menu with foods that are soft solids, semi-solids, or liquids.

Cold water or cold air always aggravates the pain, so avoid any cold beverages or foods if you have TMJ disorder. Rubbing the painful area and heat therapy always give a relief.

If you have nerve pain that comes in bouts and affects one side of your face, get yourself evaluated for trigeminal neuralgia. There is a proper medication and lifestyle regimen for this condition.

If you have pain in the jaw joint that is exaggerated by swallowing, try to eat small morsels of food at a time. Chew food very thoroughly before swallowing and take sips of water midway.

If there is constant cramping of facial muscles while eating, you may require painkillers and muscle relaxants. In that case, consult with your doctor, do some facial exercises, and take appropriate medication.

## Cures from the kitchen

Increase the general intake of fruits and vegetables in your diet. A liberal intake of fruits is beneficial in the treatment of TMJ and its allied symptoms. Fasting on an all-fruit diet is recommended because it helps clear the body of toxic radicals that cause muscular stiffness.

**'Easy-to-chew' foodstuffs** – Painful jaws require foods that are easy to chew or are semi-solids, such as soups, smoothies, and stews.

**Eat small portions of meals** – Eat only small portions of food to stabilize the blood sugar. Sporadic changes in blood sugar increase grinding of the teeth.

**Indulge in fish** – Fish contains omega 3 fatty acids can that reduce pain and inflammation in the body.

**Tons of vegetables** – Not only are they easy to chew, but there are multiple ways to enjoy various vegetables. Moreover, they are rich in nutrients that enhance healing.

**Protein shakes** – They are useful to individuals that have difficulty in chewing protein products, such as beef.

**Foods rich in magnesium** – Magnesium helps release tension in tight muscles, so it is quite useful for TMJ pain and cramps.

## Foods that TMJ patients should avoid

**Sugar products** increase inflammation and reduce the immune response.

**Caffeine** causes dehydration and increases muscular tension.

**Alcohol** hastens grinding of the teeth at night.

**Chewing gums, caramels and hard candies** worsen TMJ.

Avoid all hard foods, such as **nuts**, because they will increase the symptoms and will cause long-standing trouble if you have TMJ.

## Lifestyle adjustments

Temporomandibular joint pain can be excruciating – and it can prevent your full enjoyment of life, from eating the foods you love, to smiling, to getting the sleep you need. However, the solution to your chronic pain may not be medication or surgery. In fact, many people who suffer from TMJ pain can find relief through simple lifestyle changes. Here are six places to start:

- ☐ **Reduce your stress and anxiety.** A number of TMJ pain sufferers clench their jaws due to stress and anxiety. If this is the case with your jaw pain, you may wish to re-evaluate your life and find the root of your stress. Perhaps your pain is a sign that you need to find a better work/life balance, rest more, or seek treatment for anxiety. It is important to note that some medications used to treat depression or anxiety may make facial pain worse.

- ☐ **Stop chewing gum.** In some cases, TMJ issues are simply the results of jaw overuse. As a general rule, pain in the

TMJ or face is an indication that you should rest all of the associated muscles as much as possible. You may find that your pain fades or completely disappears when you stop chewing gum, eating hard foods, or eating crunchy foods.

☐ **Start stretching your jaw regularly.** Don't underestimate the power of simple physical therapy. Regularly stretching your jaw in the morning and evening can help keep you healthy and pain-free. Speak to your doctor about appropriate stretches for your mouth and jaw.

☐ **Eat softer, smaller pieces of food.** In addition to avoiding gum, you should watch what you eat and how you eat. Eating corn on the cob and large pieces of steak can increase TMJ pain, while eating small bites of soft foods, like mashed potatoes or soup, can give your jaw needed rest.

☐ **Don't stress your head and neck muscles.** Your jaw pain could be caused when other nearby parts of your body are stressed, such as your head and neck. Pay attention to whether stress to your neck is often paired with your TMJ disorder and whether any of your daily activities adversely affect your TMJ pain.

☐ **Confront your tooth grinding and jaw-clenching.** A significant number of TMJ pain patients find that their health issues are caused by grinding the teeth and clenching the jaw. If you believe that your TMJ disorder is related to grinding or clenching, you can take steps to control that issue. Your doctor or dentist can provide you with a custom mouth guard that will protect your jaw and teeth at night while you sleep. Use of store-bought mouth guards is not recommended, as the inappropriate design may make symptoms worse rather than better.

☐ **Wear night guards.** A night guard is a customized plastic device, usually made by a dentist that fits over your teeth and is worn at night to reduce the damage to teeth and jaw joints caused by clenching and grinding. Consult your dentist for advice on this matter.

Based on this list, people with TMJ pain suffer for a number of different reasons: some may be combating stress and anxiety, while others may suffer from teeth-grinding, neck muscle stress, or jaw abnormalities. To understand which lifestyle changes may help you combat TMJ pain, it is imperative that you understand the cause of your disorder.

## Chiropractic adjustments

Chiropractic adjustments for TMJ can help ease the pain by correcting the misalignment between the spine and nervous system. Chiropractic for TMJ can be used alone or as a complement to other treatments. The main aims of chiropractic care, in the scenario of TMJ management, are:

- ☐ Relaxing the muscles.
- ☐ Adjusting the joint.
- ☐ Using specific trigger points to reposition the jaw.

Through high-frequency, low-impact chiropractic adjustments, patients with TMJ can see improvement in the distance they can open their jaws with a decrease in pain. Many patients who have been treated for TMJ with chiropractic adjustments report relief and satisfaction.

Chiropractic treatment helps relieve pain in the short term and prevent TMJ pain from returning. Chiropractic adjustments for TMJ focus on relieving tension in the muscles around the joints using massage and trigger point therapy. Chiropractors can manipulate trigger points to relieve the pain associated with them, which is common in treating TMJ.

Adjustments to the jaw joint are done by hand when treating TMJ with chiropractic care. This technique causes a tiny stretch inside the joint to release any fibrous attachments made by the body due to previous trauma. TMJ caused by misalignment in the neck and upper back can find relief from spinal joint adjustments in these areas. Chiropractors can also use massage to minimize stress put on the jaw so other adjustments can be more effective.

By employing these treatments, the motion of the jaw joint, ear pain, jaw locking, headaches, and neck pain can be reduced. By treating the cause of the pain and discomfort associated with TMJ, chiropractic care can help reduce symptoms, which makes for a happier and less painful life. In addition to regular chiropractic treatment for TMJ, the chiropractor may also give you home exercises to strengthen the joint and muscles surrounding it.

Chiropractic adjustments for TMJ may be the solution you're looking for to stop the pop and relieve the pain associated with the disorder.

# Other alternatives therapies

## Exercises for TMJ pain relief

TMJ exercises help fortify the joints and relax the jaw. They also promote healing of the jaw. Temporomandibular joints are used daily. These TMJ joints connect the jawbone to the skull and TMJ symptoms appear when talking, chewing, and swallowing.

TMJ symptoms arise when something happens with the jaw joint and muscles. Occasionally, this scenario occurs due to injury to the jaw or inflammation caused by either arthritis or overuse of the mouth.

Temporomandibular joint disorders cause gentle to devastating symptoms, such as:

☐ Headaches;

- ☐ Jaw joint locking;

- ☐ Pain during chewing;

- ☐ Pain in the jaw, neck, face, and the ear.

- ☐ Grating, clicking, and popping sounds produced in the jaw when closing or opening the mouth.

The *Journal of Dental Research* in 2010 stated that conducting TMJ exercises enhances the mouth opening as compared to using the mouth guard, especially in people with TMJ displacement. Some of the exercises that are frequently recommended are:

## Relaxing jaw exercise

Patients should rest their tongue lightly at the top of their mouth behind their upper front teeth. They should allow teeth to appear separately while relaxing their jaw muscles.

## Goldfish exercises for partial opening

This exercise involves placing the tongue at the top of the mouth, and one finger on the ear where TMJ is situated. Place the pointer finger on the chin. The lower jaw is dropped halfway and closed immediately. Mild resistance is experienced but no pain exists. Exercise is done six times to complete one set. Patients should attempt one set daily for six times.

## Goldfish exercises for full opening

This exercise is done by keeping the tongue at the top of patient's mouth while placing one finger on the TMJ and another finger on the chin. Individuals should drop their lower jaw entirely. For a complete variation, this exercise should entail placing one finger at each TMJ while they completely drop their lower jaw. This exercise should be done six times to finish a single set. One should do a set six times daily.

## Jaw tucks

In this exercise, the patient's shoulders are pushed back and the chest is in a popping-up position. The chin is pulled back straight, forming a "double chin" that he/she holds on for at least 3 seconds and repeat it 10 times.

## Resisting mouth opening

The patient should place a thumb under the chin and open the mouth slowly, thus pushing it gently against their chin to resist. They should hold on for at least 3 to 6 seconds, after which they should close their mouth slowly.

## Resisting mouth opening in a variable position

One should squeeze the chin with both index finger and thumb of the same hand. Close the mouth, then place light pressure on the chin. This helps to strengthen muscles, which aids in chewing.

## Tongue up

While the tongue is pointing to the roof of the mouth, gradually open and close the mouth.

## Sideways jaw movement

This exercise entails placing a 14-inch object, e.g., a stacking tongue depressor, in between the teeth and moving the jaw swiftly sideways. While the process seems to be easy, add the thickness of the objects in between the teeth as you stack them on top of one another.

## Forward jaw movement

This exercise is done by placing a 4-inch object, e.g., a stacking tongue depressor, in between the teeth and moving the bottom jaw swiftly in a forward position to enable the bottom teeth to be in front of the top teeth. While the process seems to be easy, add the thickness of the objects in between the teeth as you stack them on top of one another.

# Adjustments to diet

## TMJ diet treatment

Changes in diet also help in relieving pain problems of TMJ. This section focuses on dietary changes that help manage TMJ.

- ☐ Patients with TMJ should control the ingestion of salicylates. Large consumption of salicylates blocks Vitamin K, causing anemic deficiencies.

- ☐ TMJ patients should cut back on consumption of whole grains, such as wheat and dairy products.

- ☐ Avoid food with high supplements, such as artificially supplemented Vitamin C or iron.

- ☐ TMJ patients should avoid large intake of sugar, yeast, and preservatives.

- ☐ Patients with TMJ should control the intake of fatty foods, i.e., consume the only moderate amount of saturated fats.

- ☐ TMJ patients are advised to ingest more red meat for intake of zinc, iron, and vitamins.

- ☐ Eating organ meat helps boost micronutrients that might play a role in improving the wellness of TMJ.

- ☐ Frequent ingestion of vegetable soup, with a large assortment of beans for magnesium, meat, and broth made from parts of the animal (such as bones and tendons) is a great option.

## Seeing your doctor, when and why?

For health purposes, everyone should have a regular dental checkup, since oral health is directly related to overall health. A regular dental cleaning, such as teeth cleaning at least every six months, greatly affects your overall health.

The first time a patient visits a dental hygiene department to have their teeth cleaned, he/she receives much more than just basic "cleaning." First, the healthcare provider begins with a complete periodontal chart – a baseline evaluation of the condition for each of the teeth and soft tissue. That gives a reference and, at least once a year thereafter, another checkup is required to evaluate overall oral health.

Using state-of-the-art digital equipment, this chart is stored electronically with other vital information, such as x-rays and intra-oral photographs, as part of the dental cleaning procedure. Periodontal charting evaluates the patient's gingival health, identifying "pockets" between the gums and teeth where disease and germs can multiply. Moreover, screening helps patients to avoid periodontal diseases that can cause the loss of the supporting bone, ligaments, and soft tissue around the teeth. This periodontal destruction can be caused by bacteria through plaque or calculus (tartar) accumulation, smoking, diabetes, or other health problems or genetics. Also known as gum disease, periodontal disease can greatly increase your risk of heart attack or stroke.

Because dental health is related to overall health, patients should receive an evaluation of their medical history at all dental appointments. This will include listing any new or past medical concerns (for example, hypertension or joint replacement) with a listing of all medications taken. Physicians should monitor blood pressure, not only to decrease the risk of medical emergencies, but also in relation to the patient's overall systemic health.

Once the gingival health is assessed through the periodontal charting, physicians are able to tailor the type of dental cleaning required.

A typical adult/child prophylaxis or cleaning is most often used for a patient who has healthy gums and no signs of periodontal disease.

For a patient with active periodontal disease, a deeper cleaning called "scaling and root planing (SCRP)" is required. Completed on a patient who has active periodontal disease, SCRP is designed to achieve soft tissue reattachment of the gingival ligaments to the tooth, lessening those "pockets" of infection and germs. This procedure is done comfortably much like a regular tooth cleaning in order to save both tooth loss and restore healthy systemic state.

After performing dental hygiene, physicians decide what radiographs (x-rays) should be taken. Radiographs let the doctor look for any dental decay or abnormalities in the mouth. X-rays are taken on a case-by-case basis, depending on what is best for the individual. Low-radiation digital x-rays are first to be employed to provide the doctor a clear picture of one's dental health.

Periodic checkups also include careful examinations of teeth, tongue, and gums, as well as x-rays. If the dentist finds a problem area, he/she will take time to carefully explain what the patient might need and discuss a care plan. In addition, all patients should receive an oral cancer screening at their appointments. This screening evaluates all the soft tissue in the mouth, such as the cheeks and tongue. Furthermore, the hygiene department should offer fluoride treatments for strong, healthy teeth, which are sometimes recommended, on a case-by-case basis.

A regular dental checkup not only keeps your oral health at par, but will also ward off any ensuing signs of TMJ disorder. Clearly, visiting a dentist means getting your maxillary health fully evaluated. This will be a great chance for every individual to prevent TMJ disorder most easily, instead of staying home and letting the condition get worse without an active management plan.

## Preventing future complications and disability

Complications with disability can be prevented by the use of pain relievers like ibuprofen and acetaminophen for TMJ pain. In case of severe pain, muscle relaxers might be prescribed; in certain cases, dentists might recommend the use of:

☐ Mouth guards, to prevent grinding of the teeth and clenching of the jaw; they may also aid in realigning the jaw.

☐ Warm towels to relax the ailing part.

- ☐ Ice blocks, for not more than 15 minutes per hour.

- ☐ Stress-relieving methods, to avert behaviors which cause tension in the jaw.

- ☐ Acupuncture to release the pressure in the affected area.

- ☐ Surgical intervention, when appropriate and unavoidable.

Extreme pain agitated by joints that are damaged usually call for more diverse invasive therapeutics, i.e., injections of corticosteroid into the temporomandibular joint. Generally, surgery should be regarded as a last resort.

Management of TMJ pain can be adopted with simple lifestyle changes. Patients might wish to:

- ☐ ingest soft foodstuffs to enable the TMJ to relax.

- ☐ avoid chewing hard objects.

- ☐ avoid biting nails.

- ☐ practice a good sitting posture.

- ☐ limit the size of the jaw movement, i.e., yawning.

The next chapter provides a happy ending to this journey of pain and discomfort, as you will learn how to stay happy with TMJ disorder through your lifetime with smart techniques that will be indispensable to you in your daily life.

# Chapter 05: Living happily with TMJ

## Living with TMD: A lifelong challenge

Living with TMJ disorders is a lifelong challenge for many sufferers. For many, primarily women, the constant disruption caused by the symptoms of this disorder deeply affects the quality of life. Constant pain and dysfunction coupled with dubious treatments and a lack of medical recognition have pushed many sufferers into the margins. Here are some helpful tips to live successfully with TMJ:

☐ Consult with your doctor to take analgesics for pain, and psychiatric drugs for depression.

☐ Pay frequent visits to a cognitive therapist who has experience in treating chronic pain. Cognitive therapy helps to teach how to change negative thought patterns, which in turn helps treat the depression and anxiety that go along with chronic pain.

☐ Physical therapists can help break the cycle of immobility that causes an escalation of your pain levels.

☐ Develop a treatment plan with your doctor, keeping in mind that the ideal plan should address all the areas of your life that are affected.

☐ Learn coping strategies that will help you gain a sense of control over your illness. They may not take your pain away, but may get it to a level that you can deal with.

☐ Keep a TMJ pain journal as a great way to help in figuring out the patterns. Make note of what time of day it hurt the most, what activities you were doing, and when your pain level changed, if and when you were stressed, sad, angry, etc.

☐ Try relaxation techniques such as yoga and meditation.

## Curbing psychological effects

It is often difficult for family and friends to provide required support, especially in the case of an invisible illness. After corrective surgery, it is usually difficult to correct the situation by explaining the consequences due to psychological trauma that precede such actions. Here are some ways to help:

☐ Spend some quality time with loved ones. Make a conscious effort to nourish those relationships.

☐ If you can't control your illness, do take responsibility for what you can control in your life.

☐ Ask questions to empower yourself with sufficient knowledge about TMJ. People need to feel that they are helping you.

☐ Mutually decide that negative feelings you and your loved ones may have are about the illness, and not about the person. You are allowed to be angry at your illness, but don't forget that there are positive things in your life, too.

☐ Not telling anyone results in a very lonely life.

☐ Not everyone is going to "get it" because by nature we want everything to be okay. Your life has changed, and some of your relationships will too. Try not to worry about what others will think.

## Living happily with TMD

If you're living with some level of TMJ, knowing how to recognize your individual symptoms and triggers will be vital to managing your condition. Another great way is to team up with a good physician whom it always just a phone call away. Together, you can do the background work of identifying your disease pattern, its ups and downs, and generate a strategy to manage it most smoothly.

You might still have minor headaches or pain episodes that are almost resistant to pain therapy. For such situations, it is best to devise an alternative treatment plan, such as a home remedy, that will always work for you.

The idea is to know your disease in your own unique and personalized way, as TMD does not affect every person 100% similarly. Most important, avoid stress. The second best thing you can do is spend time learning what options you have and what really works for you.

In time, you will be able to chart a successful management plan that will never falter. This will ultimately lead you to a journey of living happily with TMJ disorder.

## What else can be done?

About 12% of all Americans suffer from TMJ pain. If you are among those sufferers, you will be familiar with the kind of pain that TMD causes. Although surgery and conservative treatments are the best options for treating the issue most permanently, there are alternative methods: things to do and not do when living with TMJ.

## Things to do

First, identify your needs and pay attention to take care of them. Pay close attention to TMJ pain and it causes. Be mindful of your body posture, since it can be a major factor in flaring TMJ pain in some patients. The body posture can only be corrected through daily practicing, even though it may be difficult to retain for the first few days. After many years of subconsciously mastering poor sitting habits, changing the pattern throughout the day can greatly help. Be mindful of how you relax, i.e., avoid placing your head against your hand. Be careful how you sleep. TMJ symptoms aggravate in the morning and in the evening, so your sleeping position is quite significant in preventing further pain.

TMJ patients should be conscious of what they are indulging in. Foods such as raw vegetables, corn, and raw carrots can aggravate TMJ pain for several days. TMJ patients are advised to indulge in softer foods, such as mashed potatoes, overcooked vegetables, and softer breads, to prevent flares of pain.

## Things not to do

TMJ patients should not cover up their symptoms and pain by constantly taking painkillers. Painkillers are useful on a short-term basis but, in some cases, they tend not to work at all. Such painkillers can worsen pain for a very long period of time. Therefore, it is prudent to seek diagnosis and treatment from a qualified doctor.

Habits, such as nail biting, chewing the cap of a pen, eating ice, and unnecessary stressful acts to the jaw and teeth should be avoided at all cost. The use of hard-textured items increases TMJ pain and even worsens underlying tissues due to poor movement of the jaw.

Avoid clenching your teeth and jaw. TMJ patients under stress and anxiety and with poor body habits often exert a lot of force in their jaws, thus exacerbating TMJ pain. During the day, always keep the teeth open and apart, and relax the tongue and the lips together.

These simple and basic tasks that help improve life for TMD patients, despite considering treatment as the ultimate solution.

## The cycle of chronic pain and depression

A good first step is to visit a neuromuscular dentist who is experienced in treating TMD. This professional will discuss and evaluate your symptoms, at first seeking non-invasive ways to treat your condition. Some patients experience complete pain relief from the treatment their neuromuscular dentist provides and from the peace of mind that comes from having their condition diagnosed and treated.

Other patients need to work with their neuromuscular dentist along with another specialist, such as a psychological counselor, to find complete relief. It is important to identify and isolate the actual causes with a medical professional who has been trained to assess both issues separately and to establish the connection so that you can resolve chronic pain and gain the tools that will help you live a happy life again.

# Three exercises for living happily with TMD

Individuals living with TMD should conduct the following exercises daily to live happily with the disorder;

- ☐ A warm-up involving repetition of small mouth opening and closing movements;

- ☐ Slow stretching of the mandible, using the fingertips to pull in a downward motion; and

- ☐ Holding the stretched position for 30 seconds, repeating the stretch-and-hold process three times.

As with any exercise routine, patients should follow a doctor-recommended approach. Depending on a patient's diagnosis, most dentists may suggest stretching or strengthening exercises as part of the overall TMJ treatment plan.

## Other physical therapies

Physical therapy is commonly prescribed for patients with TMJ disorder, both as a conservative treatment and after TMJ surgery. Physical therapy is a non-invasive treatment that aims to relax muscles, improve posture, and relieve jaw pain.

On the first visit, the physical therapist will do a review of your medical history, including any surgical procedures. He or she will ask you to move the TMJ and will note any issues. This will allow the therapist to form a plan for your care. Many different treatment modalities can be performed by a physical therapist. Often, a combination of many treatments will be used.

## Physical therapy options:

☐ **TENS**: Electrical current can be applied to the TMJ area to relieve stiffness and pain.

☐ **Ultrasound**: High-frequency sound waves are transferred to the body via a round probe. The sound waves travel into the muscle to generate gentle heat.

☐ **Iontophoresis**: A non-invasive method by which medications (usually steroids and/or lidocaine) can be delivered through the skin.

☐ **Stretching Exercises**

☐ **Moist heat**: Hot packs that increase blood flow, reduce spasm, and relax muscles.

☐ **Cold Packs**: They help control inflammation, reducing spasms and pain.

☐ **Massage**: Different types of massages may be used to reduce pain and relax muscles.

☐ **Posture/Ergonomics/Sleeping**: Many physical therapists include lessons on posture, ergonomics, and sleeping positions in their sessions.

Physical therapy is a non-invasive treatment for TMJ disorder that may relax muscles, improve posture, and relieve pain. A doctor or dentist can prescribe physical therapy for TMJ disorder and some insurance companies may cover it. Many oral surgeons also prescribe a regimen of physical therapy after TMJ surgery to regain function of the jaw.

In addition, other health practitioners may suggest a variety of therapeutic treatments to reduce discomfort and promote healing.

- ☐ Apply a heat pack or hot water bottle wrapped in a lightly moistened towel to the affected area to relax tight muscles and alleviate pain. Use caution when applying heat to avoid burns.

- ☐ Wrap an ice pack in a dry cloth and hold it against the affected area to decrease inflammation and numb pain. Cold therapy should only be used for 10 to 15 minutes at a time.

- ☐ Deep, slow-breathing meditation can aid in relaxing the jaw and managing pain. Yoga or guided meditation can reduce stress and improve awareness of habits like jaw-clenching or teeth- grinding that contribute to TMJ discomfort.

- ☐ Massage therapy can relax muscle tissue, helping to lessen spasms and easing nerve compression.

- ☐ Use of over-the-counter pain medicine, such as ibuprofen, can provide temporary relief when TMJ symptoms flare up. In addition, dentists may prescribe muscle relaxers or other medications to treat ongoing spasms and pain.

Every TMJ patient is unique. The best way is to work through a trial-and-error method to identify which exercises and treatment options work best for you to decrease your pain and discomfort.

# Hope for the future

## Hormonal pathogenesis

The higher prevalence of TMJ in women is accounted for by reproductive age. Many research studies assume that sex-based determinants, such as hormonal changes, i.e., estrogen and progesterone, increase the chance of an individual contracting degenerative diseases such as TMJ. Various studies have been postulated as evidence to support this assumption, while others have refuted it. Recently, a study was done to support this notion. The researchers carried out an experiment where estrogen and progesterone were restricted in the TMJ of rats and mice of both genders and compared it with humans. The findings suggested dimorphism in sex due to the presence of estrogen receptors.

Other studies tied estrogen directly with TMJ disorders. Some of the evidence for the link suggests an association between the facial pain and estrogen replacement therapy. That is, oral contraceptive use with a systemic elevation of estrogen level in women suffering from TMJ versus those in a control group. Additionally, polymorphism contained in estrogen receptor correlates with the intensity of the axis angle in the facial pain and mandibular length of the body in patients who suffer from TMJ osteoarthritis.

A potential relationship has also been established between modulated hormonal imbalance and degradation. Moreover, this imbalance increases matrix degradation and primarily aids in the progression of the joint disease. The modified hormone-mediated changes influence the ability of the joint to maintain normal function, which can increase progressive degenerative changes in the joint. All these findings are useful in suggesting that sex hormones explicitly predispose many people to TMJ degenerations.

## Systemic and local biomarkers of disease

Biomarkers of diseases are a highly sought-after approach for the early diagnosis of various conditions and for evaluating the efficacy of treatment modalities. Various sources of samples are used for the assaying of disease biomarkers. In the case of joint disorders, these samples have included synovial lavages or aspirates, tissue samples, serum or plasma, or urine. The most common sample used in studies performed to date is synovial lavage to determine the changes in various local biological mediators of disease that may be used subsequently in predicting the status of the disease.

Findings from such studies have demonstrated increased levels of inflammatory mediators in patients with TMJ disorders versus controls. While the synovial lavage or aspirate samples are typically obtainable from subjects undergoing arthrocentesis (joint aspiration), their availability for routine diagnostics is questionable because of the invasive nature of the procedure. Also, inherent limitations in the methodology, including unknown dilution effects, make it difficult to compare data between subjects and over time and diminish the utility of this approach for diagnostic purposes.

Synovial tissues from patients with TMJ disorders are also used to evaluate potential biomarkers. Investigators using these samples have shown that there is increased expression of IL-8 and microvessel density in TMD patients. However, similar to synovial fluid, the invasiveness of the procedure to obtain samples makes the evaluation of synovial tissues less than ideal. A less invasive sampling involves assays on urine or serum.

88

Assays on urine samples have shown elevated levels of pyridinoline (Pyr) and deoxypyridinoline (Dpyr) collagen cross-links, which are known markers of bone and cartilage turnover, in patients with osteoarthritis of the TMJ.

Additionally, elevated amino acid secretion products were found in the urine of patients with chronic muscle pain TMD. Similarly, preliminary studies using serum have suggested increased estrogen levels in TMD patients and increased levels of interleukin-1 beta and C-reactive protein in arthritic TMJ diseases. No studies have been done to assay for potential biomarkers of TMJ disorders using saliva, which would be a highly desirable source for assaying biomarkers for disease or therapeutic outcomes. Also, while the studies cited above provide insights into potential biomarkers of TMJ diseases, much work remains to be done to demonstrate the specificity and sensitivity of any given marker of the disease status.

While a "gold standard" biomarker for TMJ disorders remains elusive, powerful new technologies such as microarrays on tissue, synovial fluid, and serum samples may enable the identification of specific and sensitive biomarkers of TMJ disease in the future.

Microarrays permit the analysis of the expression of thousands of genes even with extremely small quantities of sample. Therefore, the use of microarrays on blood samples from patients with TMJ disorders may be able to identify novel genes or combinations of genes that are predictive of TMDs.

In a recent study, microarray analysis of 3,543 genes in blood samples in patients with mild knee osteoarthritis and non-symptomatic controls revealed nine genes considered to be predictive of knee osteoarthritis. These nine genes were then used to blindly evaluate a new sample of 67 subjects and demonstrated

72 percent sensitivity and 66 percent specificity as a test for osteoarthritis.

In the next few years, it is likely that tests based on findings from such studies will become commercially available as viable tools to aid the clinician in the early and specific diagnosis of various joint disorders, including those involving the TMJ. Studies such as these are also likely to help identify key pathways and bioactive molecules that contribute to the perpetuation of the disease that can be targeted for rational therapeutics.

## Tissue engineering

Recent advances have been made in the field of TMD involving tissue engineering. A study conducted in Shanghai used the deep circumflex iliac artery flap with costochondral graft as a safe and dependable bone flap. The combination was used to for routine reconstruction or the mandibular body as well as the TMJ.

The procedure involves insertion of the rib into the iliac crest as a whole transplant and a fix at the proximal stump of the mandible with a pre-bent reconstruction plate in accordance with the computer-aided design. The results were amazing since the grafts healed uneventfully. The dental implants were inserted later on. The follow-up also showed that the patients had a perfect mandible function, including opening the mouth, force biting, and occlusion. From this research, the deep circumflex iliac artery flap (DCIA flap) combined with a costochondral graft is a secure and dependable method to present not only a large bulk of bone to ensemble the mandible but also the function of the TMJ.

Currently, researchers at Columbia University Medical Center have succeeded in repairing the degenerated TMJ cartilage of the mouse. This is an exciting achievement of transplanting a single stem cell. The mouse stem cell was undifferentiated into immature cells, which can potentially be converted to any form and type of the tissue in the body. This process of manipulation stem cells is a major breakthrough in science and medicine since it encourages new cell growth that can be used to treat degenerated tissue.

Furthermore, this technique can overcome the problem of the inherent risk in transplanting stem cells where the donor cells are rejected by the recipient's immune system. Colombian researchers provided an alternative approach where they manipulate the stem therapy that already exists in the area, and then they induce it to repair the tissue that is damaged.

## Using technology and biomedicine to engineer the TMJ

For many people suffering from severe and painful degenerative diseases of the TMJ, surgical replacement of the mandibular condyle remains the only option. Until recently, the primary methods employed to reconstruct the TMJ included autogenous tissue grafting, for example from the rib, or the use of alloplastic materials, with neither being ideally suited for the task and sometimes leading to extremely deleterious effects.

Fortunately, due to recent advances in the understanding of stem cell biology and biomaterials, it seems that, in the near future, it may be possible to successfully reconstruct a bioengineered TMJ replacement that is compatible with a host and biologically viable, and that can easily withstand or tolerate the physiologic loads required of this joint.

Tissue engineering involves developing, in vitro and/or in vivo, a biological replacement that mimics the biological, morphological, and organizational characteristics of the tissue it is replacing. The most common method for deriving engineered tissues involves the implantation of cells, typically derived from the host, into a biomimetic scaffold and then stimulating it in a bioreactor or in vivo with appropriate signals to develop a replacement tissue or organ. Cells from various sources, including articular cartilage cells, fibroblasts, human umbilical cord matrix stem cells, and mesenchymal stem cells, have been used in efforts to reconstruct the TMJ.

Of these cells, stem cells have gained increasing prominence in the tissue engineering of joints and have been used by various investigators for developing prototype TMJ condyles. Unlike primary cells, such as chondrocytes, that have limited capacity to propagate, stem cells have the additional advantage of being stimulated by specific biological cues into differentiating into osteoblasts, chondrocytes, fibroblasts, and myocytes. These cell types, in turn, generate cartilage, bone, ligaments, and muscles, respectively, to derive all key components of the TMJ complex. Thus, for example, in recent studies, rat bone marrow mesenchymal stem cells were grown separately in chondrogenic differentiation media or in osteoblastic differentiation media. Subsequent transfer of the two cell populations into a scaffold with two stratified and integrated layers, and then implantation into the backs of immunodeficient mice for 12 weeks, resulted in a structure containing both cartilage and bone tissue in a construct with the shape and dimensions of the human mandibular condyle.

# Current advancements

## Physical therapy

Physical therapy advancements have enabled stretching of the jaw and relaxing temporomandibular joints as well as the muscles around it. Physical therapy also helps with soft tissue stretching, joint movement, posture, and the upper cervical spine.

Physical therapy is an effective method adopted by most doctors. Moreover, most dentists worldwide recommend the therapy to most patients. Advanced technology use for TMJ treatment can identify the fundamental causes and symptoms of TMD. Furthermore, this method helps all the stakeholders to establish customized treatment programs that address each area for relief purposes.

The main objective of advanced therapy is the improvement of alignment and mobility through exercise and manual therapy that reduces the load on the TMJ, thus increasing flexibility and strengthening the muscles. When a patient is suffering from an injury or has previously had a surgery, scar tissue is released by physical therapy. The use of ultrasound and electrical stimulation tools is also implemented to decrease the pain.

## TENS

A transcutaneous nerve stimulation (TENS) device employs mild electrical currents that are passed through the skin over the jaw muscles. It helps to block pain signals, thus increasing blood circulation and relaxation of the muscles.

# Ultrasound therapy

This device utilizes sound waves of higher frequencies by directing them to the TMJ joint. Ultrasound sound waves reduce the swelling and improve circulation while decreasing the pain.

Ultrasound therapy is used as an adjunct modality for the treatment of pain in the head and neck. It uses very high-frequency sound waves to stimulate the tissue beneath the skin's surface. The energy is primarily absorbed by connective tissue, such as ligaments, tendons, and fascia. This tissue can be treated in the jaw, neck, and shoulder area for relief of pain associated with temporomandibular disorders.

**Features of ultrasound therapy**

- Relief from pain and joint contractures that may be associated with:
  - Adhesive capsulitis
  - Bursitis with slight calcification
  - Myositis
  - Soft tissue injuries
  - Shortened tendons due to past injuries and scar tissues
- Relief from sub-chronic and chronic pain, and joint contractures resulting from:
  - Capsular tightness
  - Capsular scarring

# Photomodulation (low-level laser therapy)

Low-level light therapy is used an adjunct modality for the treatment of pain in the head and neck. The use of applied photons on deep tissues can increase tissue repair, muscle relaxation, and pain control. The therapy is non-invasive and effective, without generating heat or the use of medication. The machine is cleared, so long as it provides pure infrared laser energy for the many indications.

**Objectives of cold laser therapy**

- ☐ Increase in local blood circulation
- ☐ Relief of minor muscle and joint aches, pains and stiffness
- ☐ Relaxation of muscles
- ☐ Temporary relief of muscle spasms
- ☐ Temporary relief of minor pain and stiffness associated with arthritis

## TENS

This technology involves the use of controlled low-voltage electrical impulses transmitted through the skin for relief of pain. TENS can reduce pain by inhibiting nociceptive receptors at the presynaptic dorsal horn of the spinal cord. Electrical stimulation through the skin preferentially activates low threshold myelinated nerve fibers, blocking transmission of pain signals from the unmyelinated fibers.

**Indications for TENS therapy includes:**

- ☐ Neurogenic pain
  - o Differentiation pain
  - o Phantom pain
  - o Sympathetically mediated pain
  - o Post-herpetic neuralgia
  - o Trigeminal neuralgia
  - o Atypical facial pain

- Musculoskeletal pain
  - Arthralgia resulting from rheumatoid arthritis or osteoarthritis
  - Chronic myofascial pain

## Electrotherapy

Electrogalvanic stimulation (EGS) technology for TMJ is used as adjunctive therapy for patients with musculoskeletal problems. It works by producing a low average current to help with treatment of muscle spasms, edema, decreased blood flow, and the location and treatment of myofascial trigger points.

**Electrotherapy features:**

- Clinical protocols for acute pain
- Chronic pain
- Increased localized circulation
- Preventing or retarding disuse muscle atrophy
- Muscle re-education
- Joint range of motion

As with other areas of medicine and dentistry, advances in biomedicine and computer-based technologies offer great promise for helping patients predisposed to or suffering from TMJ diseases. These technologies will enhance diagnostic capabilities and rational therapeutics or preventive strategies. Genetic analysis, biomarkers, imaging, and tissue engineering will likely expand the repertoire and improve the specificity of diagnostic and therapeutic approaches for diseases of the TMJ. Progress in biomedicine, imaging, and computer technology also point to the need for academicians, researchers, and the healthcare community to appropriately educate and prepare future clinicians to take advantage of these innovations.

# Conclusion

The TMJ is one of the most-used joints in the human body and, sadly, this joint is also the most underrated in terms of its safety indications, management, and treatment. More than 12% of U.S. residents have some form of TMJ disorder, whether it's due to bad chewing habits, excessive and aggressive usage, or an underlying pathology.

This eBook is your ultimate guide to understanding TMJ disorder with a holistic approach. We have armed you with all the knowledge and understanding you need to get to know your condition and find the most suitable management plan. We have also including some precious home remedies and life hacks that will make living with TMD a breeze.

We wish you luck on your journey to battle this issue with confidence, and we hope that this eBook serves as a pioneer in helping you in your journey.

Feel free to come back and re-read your favorite or most important parts. Share this treasure with a loved one who needs help or keep it with you as a reference guide that is evergreen in its science-backed knowledge and is a helpful friend in your times of pain and discomfort.

# References

1. Dıraçoğlu, Demirhan, et al. (2016). Temporomandibular dysfunction and risk factors for anxiety and depression. *Journal of Back and Musculoskeletal Rehabilitation*, 29.3, 487-491.

2. Müller, L., van Waes, H., Langerweger, C., Molinari, L., & Saurenmann, R. K. (2013). Maximal mouth opening capacity: percentiles for healthy children 4–17 years of age. *Pediatric Rheumatology*, 11(1), 17.

3. Craft, R. M. (2007). Modulation of pain by estrogens. *Pain,* 132, S3-S12.

4. Chisnoiu, A. M., Picos, A. M., Popa, S., Chisnoiu, P. D., Lascu, L., Picos, A., & Chisnoiu, R. (2015). Factors involved in the etiology of temporomandibular disorders: a literature review. *Clujul Medical*, 88(4), 473.

5. Ferrazzo, K. L., Osorio, L. B., & Ferrazzo, V. A. (2013). CT images of a severe TMJ osteoarthritis and differential diagnosis with other joint disorders. *Case Reports in Dentistry*, 2013.

6. Brooks, SL, et al. (1997) Imaging of the temporomandibular joint. Position paper of the American Academy of Oral and Maxillofacial Radiology. *Oral Surg Oral Med Oral Pathol Oral Radiol Endod*, 83:609.

7. Gerards, M. (2015). Musculoskeletal ultrasound of the temporomandibular joint muscles. Retrieved from http://sharing-

science.com/images/fontys/speakers/Marissa_Gerards/The
sis%20v1.0%20Marissa%20Gerards.pdf

8. Melis, M., Secci, S., & Ceneviz, C. (2007). Use of ultrasonography for the diagnosis of temporomandibular joint disorders: a review. *Am J Dent, 20*(2), 73-78.

9. Wright, E. F., Clark, E. G., Paunovich, E. D., & Hart, R. G. (2006). Headache improvement through TMD stabilization appliance and self-management therapies. *CRANIO®, 24*(2), 104-111.

10. Daynes, E., & Horgan, T. (2015). Physiotherapists prescribing non-steroidal anti-inflammatory drugs and analgesics. *Physiotherapy, 101*, e302-e303.

*11.* Gauer, R. L., & Semidey, M. J. (2015). Diagnosis and treatment of temporomandibular disorders. *American Family Physician, 91*(6).

12. Beecroft, E. V., Durham, J., & Thomson, P. (2013). Retrospective examination of the healthcare 'journey' of chronic orofacial pain patients referred to oral and maxillofacial surgery. *British Dental Journal, 214*(5), E12-E12.

13. Bradley, P. F. (1987). Conservative treatment for temporomandibular joint pain dysfunction. *British Journal of Oral and Maxillofacial Surgery, 25*(2), 125-137.

14. Dutt, C. S., Ramnani, P., Thakur, D., & Pandit, M. (2015). Botulinum toxin in the treatment of muscle specific pro-facial pain: a literature review. *Journal of maxillofacial and oral surgery, 14*(2), 171-175.

15. Gonzalez-Perez, L. M., Infante-Cossio, P., Granados-Nunez, M., Urresti-Lopez, F. J., Lopez-Martos, R., & Ruiz-Canela-Mendez, P. (2015). Deep dry needling of

trigger points located in the lateral pterygoid muscle: efficacy and safety of treatment for management of myofascial pain and temporomandibular dysfunction. *Medicina Oral, Patologia Oral y Cirugia Bucal, 20*(3), e326.

16. Messina, G., Martines, F., Thomas, E., Salvago, P., Fabris, G. B. M., Poli, L., & Iovane, A. (2017). Treatment of chronic pain associated with bruxism through myofunctional therapy. *European Journal of Translational Myology*, 27(3).

17. Zhang, S., Yap, A. U., & Toh, W. S. (2015). Stem cells for temporomandibular joint repair and regeneration. *Stem Cell Reviews and Reports, 11(5), 728-742.*

18. Lakshman, A. R., Babu, G. S., & Rao, S. (2015). Evaluation of effect of transcutaneous electrical nerve stimulation on salivary flow rate in radiation induced xerostomia patients: a pilot study. *Journal of Cancer Research and Therapeutics, 11*(1), 229.

19. Rodrigues, D., Siriani, A. O., & Bérzin, F. (2004). Effect of conventional TENS on pain and electromyographic activity of masticatory muscles in TMD patients. *Brazilian Oral Research*, 18(4), 290-295.

20. Gomez, C. E., & Christensen, L. V. (1991). Stimulus-response latencies of two instruments delivering transcutaneous electrical neuromuscular stimulation (TENS). *Journal of Oral Rehabilitation*, 18(1), 87-94.

21. Ueda, H. M., Kato, M., Saifuddin, M., Tabe, H., Yamaguchi, K., & Tanne, K. (2002). Differences in the fatigue of masticatory and neck muscles between male and female. *Journal of Oral Rehabilitation*, 29(6), 575-582.

22. Olate, S., Martinez, F., Uribe, F., Pozzer, L., Cavalieri-Pereira, L., & de Moraes, M. (2014). TMJ function after partial condylectomy in active mandibular condylar hyperplasia. *International Journal of Clinical and Experimental Medicine*, 7(3), 775.

23. Vibhute, P. J., Bhola, N., & Borle, R. M. (2011). TMJ ankylosis: multidisciplinary approach of treatment for dentofacial enhancement—a case report. *Case reports in dentistry*, *2011*.

24. Bulgannawar, B. A., Rai, B. D., Nair, M. A., & Kalola, R. (2011). Use of temporalis fascia as an interpositional arthroplasty in temporomandibular joint ankylosis: analysis of 8 cases. *Journal of Oral and Maxillofacial Surgery*, 69(4), 1031-1035.

25. Escoda Francolí, J., Vázquez Delgado, E., & Gay Escoda, C. (2010). Scientific evidence on the usefulness of intraarticular hyaluronic acid injection in the management of temporomandibular dysfunction. *Medicina Oral, Patología Oral y Cirugia Bucal*, 15(4), 644-648.

26. Wadhwa, S., & Kapila, S. (2008). TMJ disorders: future innovations in diagnostics and therapeutics. *Journal of Dental Education*, 72(8), 930-947.

27. Manfredini, D., Guarda-Nardini, L., & Ferronato, G. (2009). Single-needle temporomandibular joint arthrocentesis with hyaluronic acid. Preliminary data after a five-injection protocol. *Minerva stomatologica*, 58(10), 471-478

28. Aryaei, A., Vapniarsky, N., Hu, J. C., & Athanasiou, K. A. (2016). Recent tissue engineering advances for the

treatment of temporomandibular joint disorders. *Current Osteoporosis Reports*, 14(6), 269-279.

CPSIA information can be obtained
at www.ICGtesting.com
Printed in the USA
BVOW09s1752130318
510477BV00011B/190/P